Joan Lunden's
Healthy Living

Joan Lunden's Healthy Living

A Practical, Inspirational Guide to Creating Balance in Your Life

JOAN LUNDEN AND LAURA MORTON

Crown Publishers, Inc.
New York

Published by Crown Publishers, Inc., 201 East 50th Street, New York, New York 10022. Member of the Crown Publishing Group.

Random House, Inc. New York, Toronto, London, Sydney, Auckland

http://www.randomhouse.com/

CROWN is a trademark of Crown Publishers, Inc.

Printed in the United States of America

Design by Maggie Hinders

Library of Congress Cataloging-in-Publication Data

Lunden, Joan.

[Healthy living]

Joan Lunden's healthy living: a practical, inspirational guide to creating balance in your life / by Joan Lunden and Laura Morton.

Includes bibliographical references

1. Women—Health and hygiene. 2. Women—Mental health. I. Title

RA778.L949   1997
96-39677

613'.0424—dc21
CIP

ISBN 0-517-70895-7

10 9 8 7 6 5 4 3 2 1

First Edition

p. 15 (right) © Alan Wanzenberg; p. 16 © 1995 Outline Press Syndicate, Inc./Timothy White; p. 20 © ABC-TV/Ida Mae Astute; p. 22 © 1996 ABC-TV/George Lange; pp. 25, 58, 78, 138, 142, 146, 148, 151, 189, 202, 205, 212, 214, 220, 237 © 1996 New Life Entertainment/Simon Bruty; pp. 26, 29 printed courtesy of the Golden Door; p. 31 © 1995 Scott Frances/Esto; pp. 34, 132 © 1996 New Life Entertainment/Larry Busacca; p. 52© 1996 ABC-TV; p. 53 Reprinted from *Make the Connection: Ten Steps to a Better Body and a Better Life* by Bob Greene and Oprah Winfrey. Copyright © 1996 Harpo, Inc., and Bob Greene and Oprah Winfrey. Reprinted with permission by Hyperion.; p. 57 © 1994 The White House; p. 61 Joan Lunden personal collection/Bob Cass; pp. 64, 95, 206, 225 © 1996 ABC-TV/Andrew Eccles; p. 69 © 1996 ABC-TV/The Walt Disney Company; p. 71 © James Leslie Parker; pp. 72, 73 © 1994 Ketcham Photo/Kym Ketcham; p. 74 Joan Lunden personal collection/Larry Busacca; p. 84 © Jon Kabat-Zinn/Priscilla Harmel; p. 90 © 1980 ABC-TV/Ken Regan-Camera Five; p. 92 © 1982 ABC-TV/Joe McNally; p. 93 © 1980 ABC-TV/Ed Sorel; p. 94 © 1994 ABC-TV/Steve Fenn; p. 96 © 1996 ABC-TV/Ida Mae Astute; p. 97 © 1994 Tina Harrison/Whetstone Photography; p. 98 © ABC-TV/Fred Watkins; p. 102 © 1995 ABC-TV; p. 104 © 1996 Outline Press Syndicate, Inc./Steven Danelian; pp. 107, 172, 192, 195 © 1995 New Life Entertainment/Tom Eckerle; p. 116 © 1985 ABC-TV/Fred Watkins; p. 120 © 1996 ABC-TV/Virginia Sherwood; p. 122 © 1996 Cosmopolitan; pp. 128, 238 © 1994 Outline Press Syndicate, Inc./Timothy White; pp. 133, 134 © 1996 ABC-TV/Simon Bruty; p. 160 Jeff Konigsberg personal collection; p. 163 © Wayne Logan/Wayne Logan Photo; p. 164 © 1996 ABC-TV/George Lange; p. 180 Joan Lunden personal collection/Ben Craine; p. 182 © 1983 Jacques Silberstein; p. 186 © 1980 ABC-TV; pp. 192, 195 © 1995 New Life Entertainment/Tom Eckerle; p. 198 © Deepak Chopra/Ed Krieger; p. 199 © 1990 ABC-TV/Ida Mae Astute; p. 216 © 1994 Republic Pictures/Timothy White; pp. 226, 227, 229 © 1996 ABC-TV/Donna Svennevik; p. 230 © 1996 Annie Leibovitz/Contact; all other photographs are from Joan Lunden's personal collection

Acknowledgments

This book would not have been possible without the influence and support of my good friend and co-author, Laura Morton. She truly taught me to enjoy life again. Thank you for helping me tap into my playful side, to once again discover a lightness of spirit and a passion for life. A whole new world has opened up for me.

I also want to acknowledge some of the people who have had a tremendous impact on me over the past few years, and those who have taken their time to help me with this book. I thank them for educating and inspiring me.

On rare occasions, you read something that dramatically alters your perception of the world and of yourself. For me that is certainly true of Dr. Jon Kabat-Zinn's *Wherever You Go, There You Are.* Thank you for allowing me to tap into your wisdom, both personally and for the purpose of writing this book. Your writing has changed my life forever.

Another profound writer who has taught me to look at the world and how I exist in it in a whole new way is Dr. Deepak Chopra. You have taught me that my life is a journey not a destination—it's much more enjoyable that way, thank you!

Dr. James Rippe, well-known cardiologist and author of *Fit Over Forty,* has joined me many times on *GMA* for our ongoing fitness segments. He is someone who can explain medical information in a clear and simple way.

A special thank-you to Dr. Tim Johnson, *GMA*'s medical editor, and to Dr. Nancy Snyderman, our medical correspondent. I thank them for always keeping me up-to-date. Their contribution to *GMA* and to this book has been invaluable.

And to psychologist Dr. Ellen

McGrath, also a regular contributor on *GMA* and author of *When Feeling Bad Is Good,* special thanks for her expert advice and inspiration. She truly knows how to help all of us put things into perspective.

To nutritionist Michelle Daum and to La Palestra dietitian Ellie Krieger, thank you for helping us understand how to be good to our bodies. My body thanks you too.

A special thank-you to fitness trainer Barbara Brandt, who helped turn my life around and shape my tomorrow. And to fitness expert Pat Manocchia of La Palestra Center for Preventative Medicine: you know I'd climb tall mountains for you. I look forward to smaller thighs, bigger pecs, and higher summits.

How can I ever thank the dynamic team of Elise Silvestri and Scot Evans? It would have been impossible to finish this book under my deadline without your undying energy, enthusiasm, and nonreactive behavior. What a pleasure to be able to work on this special project with such wonderful friends. A special thanks to writer-researcher Cheryl Olsen, M.P.H., S.D., for her expertise on women's health issues.

To Jill Alpert, my assistant at *GMA,* who with her typical grace and speed became Jill Alpert Seigerman before this book was completed. I wish you happiness and joy as you enter this new cycle of life. Thank you to Sara Shields for your tireless effort seeing to the details of this book. A million thanks to makeup artist Michelle Cutler and hairstylist Kristen Barry who keep me looking my best every morning on *GMA,* not to mention the pictures in this book. Thank you also to Mark Daniel Fonzi and David Evangelista for working wonders with my hair.

To Anne Marie Riccitelli, director of media relations at ABC, where can I begin to thank you for the careful guidance and personal attention you have given me over the years at ABC. And to Peter Murray and Ida Astute in the ABC photography department, you went above and beyond helping me on this project and I will never forget it.

Thanks to Jim Wagner, vice president of marketing and promotion for *GMA,* and to Robert Pini, *GMA*'s director of public relations, for your constant support and belief in this project. And thanks to *GMA* executive producer Marc Burstein for helping me believe in myself.

And now for two men whose faith and confidence continue to inspire me to take projects like this. Marc Chamlin, my attorney, who has navigated many stormy seas and has remained my anchor over the years. He is a friend who I can trust to give me straightforward answers. And to Al Lowman, my book agent, for challenging me to go in search of new questions. His belief in me has helped me in my journey to find the answers.

Also, special thanks to everyone at the Little Dix Bay Resort in Virgin Gorda, BVI. Many of the photographs for this book were taken there, and the staff couldn't have been more accommodating.

Thanks to Debra Szekely and Ann Bernstein of the Golden Door. I'm so grateful for your cooperation and contribution to the project. And to Kip Rosenthal, my riding trainer, for her constant guidance and support.

Thanks to Lauren Shakely and Katie Workman who have to read and edit all of those questions and answers. Your leadership has helped guide this project from the start. We thank you and your team at Clarkson Potter and Crown Publishers. This experience has been a complete pleasure for me. And thanks to Chip Gibson, Andrew Martin, Barbara Marks, Maggie Hinders, Erica Youngren, Laurie Stark, Teresa Nicholas, and Amy Boorstein for all of your work.

And I could never go without thanking my mother, Gladyce Blunden, who gave me strength and self-confidence, and of course to my daughters, Jamie, Lindsay, and Sarah. You not only provide me with much love and joy in my life . . . you also provide me with a lot of good stories to tell.

Contents

Dedication

I remember the day my father died as if it were yesterday. There I was, thirteen years old, standing by the runway waving good-bye as my dad's plane lifted off the ground. He had asked my mother and my brother, Jeff, and me to accompany him on a short business trip to Los Angeles, but my mom decided that my brother and I shouldn't miss school. At the last minute she changed her mind, picked us up at school, and rushed home to catch Dad before he left. As luck would have it, just as we pulled up to the house that afternoon my father's plane was taking off down the runway that bordered our fly-in ranch. We missed him by moments. I stood there that day waving good-bye, totally unaware that this was the last time I would ever see my father. Dad's plane crashed somewhere in Malibu Canyon on his way back home. The cause of the crash was unknown, and his body was never found. For the longest time I held

on to the belief that somehow Dad was okay. I maintained a child's fantasy that he survived the crash but was left with amnesia and was now living happily somewhere else.

Although it's been years, my father's death still has a profound effect on my life. My father always told me that I could be anything I chose, but whatever I decided to be, I was to be the best at it. He used to take me on his rounds at his hospital, proudly introduce me to his patients, and talk about how someday I too would become a doctor. He was fluent in a number of languages, having been born in Australia and raised in China. His family moved to the United States during his teen years so that he could attend medical school here. His Spanish was so fluent that he often was asked to travel to Mexico to deliver medical symposiums on his specialty, which was cancer. I studied Spanish in gram-

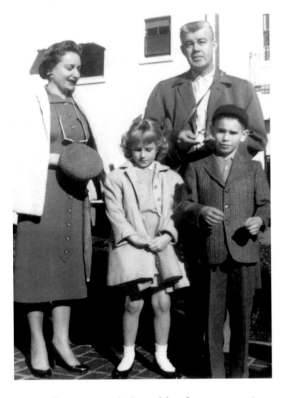

Me with my mom, dad, and brother, on vacation in 1958.

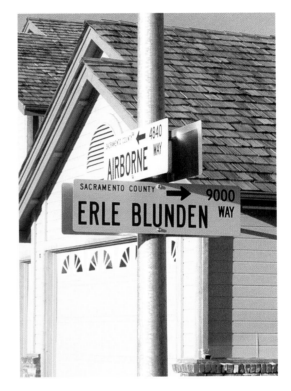

A street in Sacramento, California, was named in memory of my dad.

mar school and he took pleasure in speaking to me only in Spanish at the dinner table. I always enjoyed the challenge. Dad was the consummate educator. His words of constant encouragement ring in my ears to this very day. They are quite often my inspiration to rise above the roadblocks of life; to succeed as a parent, a worker, a friend;

and to be the best I can be. In fact, I even believe that he looks out for me as my guardian angel. My friends tell me that I must have a lucky star because somehow things seem to turn out right for me. I just smile, because I know that my lucky star is my dad watching over me.

When I was younger, I didn't realize just how much my dad meant to all the

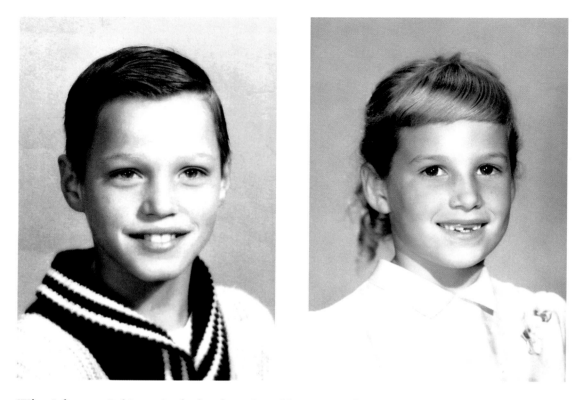

When I first met Jed I was in the fourth grade and he was "an older man" in the fifth grade.

other people whose lives he touched. He was a recognized cancer specialist who built his own hospital, where I worked part-time as a teenager. He was one of the few doctors in a fifty-mile radius surrounding Sacramento, California, so he affected thousands of lives over the years. He delivered babies, cured ailments, and saved lives. I still hear from many of his patients today.

There is another person whom I think about often, someone who also had a profound impact on my life. While growing up, two of my closest friends were twins named Jed and Jay Johnson. They were always at my house—their mom would even call us and ask if she could "borrow" the boys for dinner! In fact, Jed was my first boyfriend, and from the fourth grade until the seventh grade I only had eyes for him. The boys came on family vacations with us and even spent holidays with us. My dad was like a father to Jed and Jay. I never realized until recently just how much my father's untimely death affected Jed, something I would only learn of through Jed's own untimely death. And until that time I never realized how much I too still hurt inside.

Jed Johnson was killed in the TWA Flight 800 tragedy on July 16, 1996. I found out about Jed's death while preparing to do a live update to the West Coast the next morning. We do *Good Morning America* live every day on the East Coast. Providing that there is no breaking or ongoing news story, that same show is aired on the West Coast three hours later. On busy news mornings, however, we're quite often in the studio until noon, doing a new version of our show for the West Coast, offering last-minute updates. July 17, 1996, was one of those mornings.

Moments before we were to open the West Coast show, I received a call from Jay, who was frantically trying to confirm that Jed was on the TWA flight list. Three minutes to air, I received con-firmation through ABC News that Jed's name did in fact appear on the passenger manifest. As we opened the show that morning, I was numb with grief. I had never before, in my twenty years on *GMA,* gone on the air unable to speak, but that morning, Charlie Gibson, my co-host on *Good Morning America* for nearly eleven years, explained to the viewers that I needed a few moments to regain my composure. It seemed impossible. How could something like this happen? Jed's sudden death, like my father's, just didn't make any sense to me at all. They were not finished with their work on this earth.

In the ensuing weeks, as I reported daily on the crash and described the bodies and plane parts being brought to the surface of the Atlantic Ocean, I soon realized that Jed's death reminded me so much of losing my father. Emotions that had been tucked away deep down inside me for over thirty years were rising to the surface. At Jed's funeral, I was reunited with his entire family for the first time since 1976. His little sister, Susie, melted into my arms, sobbing. She told me that she too was reminded of the day my dad was killed. She recalled that Jed was so distraught over losing my father that he locked himself in his room for days and refused to come out and eat or speak to anyone. Thirty years later I am completely dumbfounded that I never knew how much my dad's death affected one of my closest friends. How ironic to find this out at a memorial service for Jed, who had also died in a plane crash.

Remembering my dad's constant words of encouragement to always be my best, I couldn't help but recall that if it hadn't been for Jed Johnson, I might not have come to New York to accept the job with ABC. He encouraged me and helped instill in me the belief that I could make it in the Big Apple. He even helped me find my first apartment. He introduced me to all of his friends and basically made sure that I was all right. That was over twenty years ago. The past few years we didn't see as much of each other as we once did, but we never forgot each other's birthday, and we always tried to get together around the holidays. Jed had gone on to become a very well known interior designer, running his own firm with his life partner, Alan Wanzenberg.

There is a reason why I have chosen to share these two very personal stories with you. There was a time in my life when I would have been paralyzed by the sadness I felt. But those are the emotions of a victim, and I have come to understand that there are people who come into our lives and help formulate who we become, and events that occur that will change our perspective. A terrible, tragic moment, though difficult at the time, can become a source of strength and courage. As I went through this recent sadness I was finally able to bring closure to my father's death, something I wasn't really aware of needing until Jed's funeral. But without closure it is almost impossible to heal and move forward emotionally. Instead of feeling like victims of painful events, we need to understand that those events are inevitable, and keeping a proper perspective can help us grow and gain new meaning in our lives. Allowing ourselves to experience adversity helps us face our greatest fears and overcome them. We can rise to the challenge of life's difficult moments and discover new strengths we never knew we had.

The purpose of this book is to help

you explore and identify the different stages and cycles of your life and to provide you with new ways to cope and make a happier, healthier life for yourself, physically, emotionally, and spiritually. You're in charge of your own happiness and the quality of your time on this earth. Some of us are given the opportunity to finish our work, and tragically some of us are taken way too soon. I dedicate this book to the memory of two such people. To my dad, Erle Blunden, who encouraged me always to try to be the best at whatever I chose to do. I remember every word you ever said, Dad. And to my dear friend Jed Johnson, whose devotion and support gave me the courage to pursue my dream in New York. Without you both, I would not be where I am today.

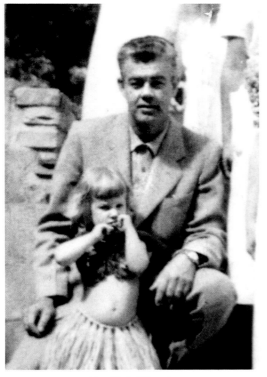

Dr. Erle Blunden
1912–1964

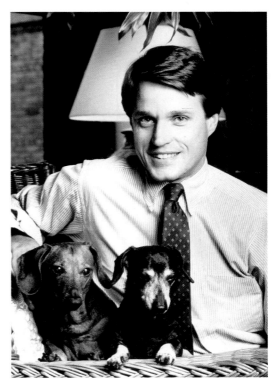

Jed Johnson
1948–1996

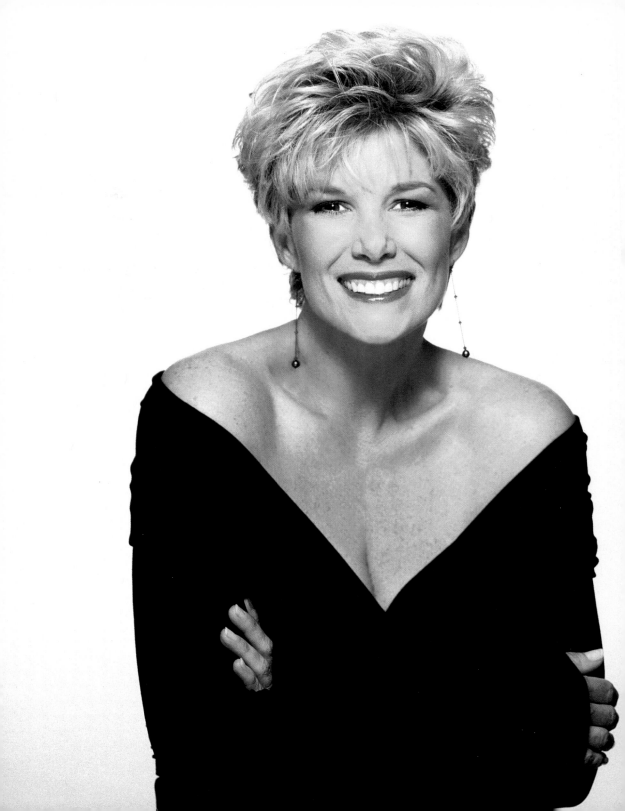

Introduction

These days, the three most asked questions of me are:

1. How have you maintained such a healthy lifestyle?

2. What's your next exciting adventure?

3. Who are you dating?

The answers are:

1. Read this book.

2. I'm climbing mountains!

3. Enough already!

Boy, has my life changed! Everywhere I go, people notice the difference in me. Not just in my physical appearance but also in my overall attitude. When I was unfit and unhealthy, I used to ask myself, "How did I get here?" It seemed that I was trapped in a place from which I couldn't escape. But I was wrong! I just had to make the *choice* to turn myself around. It certainly didn't happen by accident. This was the beginning of my own realization that we choose what we will become.

Some of the changes were easy to recognize, like my weight loss. Others were less tangible, yet equally powerful in their impact on my life. Especially the discovery of the mind-body connection. Understanding this connection can help promote better health, quicker recovery from illness, and a feeling of emotional well-being. I hope to help you discover and explore your own connection between mind and body. Once you've grasped on to the influence each has on the other, you will see that both must be nurtured and cared for in order for you to achieve total wellness.

"Health is not just the absence of a disease. It's an inner joyfulness that should be ours all the time—a state of positive well-being."
DEEPAK CHOPRA

To achieve total health, you must embrace and truly understand the importance of being in touch with your feelings. It takes self-awareness to be able to change what's making you unhappy and to achieve self-acceptance. If you take the time, this important introspective period can really transform your life. Live each day in the moment, and stop being preoccupied with your past and your future. This will help you stay focused and appreciate the joys in your life right now.

Over recent years I have witnessed how this has changed my life, and so have my friends and my family. It has been great fun for me, however, to have these changes noticed by people like you and to realize that my enthusiasm for my newfound life bubbles over enough that many of you have been influenced to change your lives too!

I wrote an article for a national women's magazine in June 1996 touching on a lot of the subjects that are discussed in this book, such as positive thinking, nonreactive behavior, and taking responsibility for your happiness. Magazines rarely send me correspondence that they receive in response to an article, so needless to say I was quite moved when they passed along the following letters from two of their readers.

HOW SHE TURNED HER LIFE AROUND

I have never written to a magazine before. I felt compelled to do so now. I am going through a very tough time in my life and it feels like it is over. I am thirty-nine. Last week I was suicidal, and after reading Joan's article I have come through it. At least I am taking it one day at a time. I hope to be able to buy her book.

I just wanted to let you know how inspiring Joan Lunden's article in your June issue was (also in hope to let Ms. Lunden know as well). Right now I'm having a difficult time at work trying to deal with an agency that is tearing itself apart as well as at home trying to get a loan for a new home. Every time something negative happens, I see it as being my problem that I need to fix. But after reading this article. things such as "a day isn't a good or bad one because of what happens around you. If you can stop reacting to events, they will no longer determine whether a day is good or bad—you will" and "You can't stop the waves, but you can learn to surf" have changed my whole perspective. Again, I just want to thank you and Ms. Lunden for the positive energy and outlook to keep me going.

While I don't profess to be an expert on mental or physical health, I do think of myself as a conduit or interpreter of information. As the host of *GMA*, "visiting" people's homes each morning, I am aware that I have an impact on my audience. These kinds of letters, whether written in response to the television show or to a magazine article, touch me in such a way that I feel compelled to continue to share what I have learned.

Again, I found the same reaction when I hosted a health and happiness series for *GMA* called *New Year, New You.* I knew that many of my viewers would make their annual New Year's resolutions to lose weight, get fit, and take charge of their own lives, just as I had for so many years in the past. This year I wanted to arm them with the latest health and fitness information to

help give them the opportunity to get a real kick start and to inspire them to begin actively participating in their own happiness. I really wanted them to feel that I was there for them.

Obviously, many of you saw those shows, because we have never received such a huge response to a series on *GMA*. I am always amazed at the number of people who write in and what they write about. Some just write to say that they love my hair, hate my shoes, or even that...they have the perfect guy for me!

Although I'm used to receiving letters, I was not prepared for the extraordinary response to the series. Thousands of letters poured in via mail, FedEx, and America Online. There were some letters simply thanking me for the inspiration. Others wrote to share their struggles or to enthusiastically declare their new commitment. Here are some of those letters.

Since I started working out, my marriage is healthier, my relationships with friends are stronger because I feel better about myself, and I just enjoy life more. It's amazing what a little self-esteem

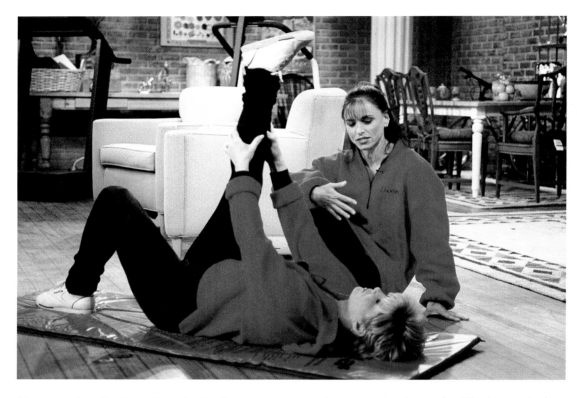

Fitness trainer Barbara Brandt showing me some proper stretching exercises for GMA's New Year, New You *series.*

can do for a gal! Thanks, GMA, for your New Year, New You *special.*

The key point I've gotten from New Year, New You *is that one must be committed to a life change, and as you have said, Joan—not to expect miracles overnight. I plan on taking classes well*

into my nineties and still plan to look and feel young at that point in my life.

I am thirty-seven years old and eighty pounds overweight. I'm a stress eater. Ten years ago I lost forty-five pounds on my own, and remember how hard it was to lose it. I kept telling myself that I was just going to like myself the way I was. Problem: I didn't like myself. With Joan as a role model, I tuned in to the GMA New Year, New You *series. I was see-*

ing myself as lean and tan, and working up a sweat and loving it! I know I can do it now. My mind is in the right place. I have made a realistic goal to lose only ten pounds in January. This week I have lost two pounds. It may be a little success in numbers, but it is a big *success emotionally.*

I am a forty-two-year-old African-American lady. I will get my life back! The life that I know I deserve. Right now I am overweight, depressed, and sad. I know it will get better. I must take control of my life. So...Ms. Lunden...I am committed to take this challenge in 1996. I am working up a real old-fashioned southern sweat!

I am a thirteen-year-old girl who has lost twenty-five pounds within the past nine months. I can tell you one thing, it hasn't been easy! It is a long, hard, and frustrating process, but well worth it! I not only feel better but look better and have more energy. Thank you, Good Morning America!

These letters are just a small sampling of what came over the World Wide Web. I was moved by each and every one. So much so that I knew my commitment to my newfound healthy lifestyle needed to be more than just a promise to myself.

Everyone I talked to about writing this book—my friends, my family, my co-workers, even my doctors—has expressed the overwhelming sentiment that I must share my wild enthusiasm. My insatiable thirst for growth had taken me into bookstore after bookstore, resulting in piles and piles of books on positive thinking, spirituality, the search for happiness, mindful focus and meditation, and every other form of self-improvement under the sun, but I was beginning to realize that the books were either too academic or way too esoteric.

Ultimately, I have decided that if you want to read a book, but it hasn't been written yet, you must write it yourself!

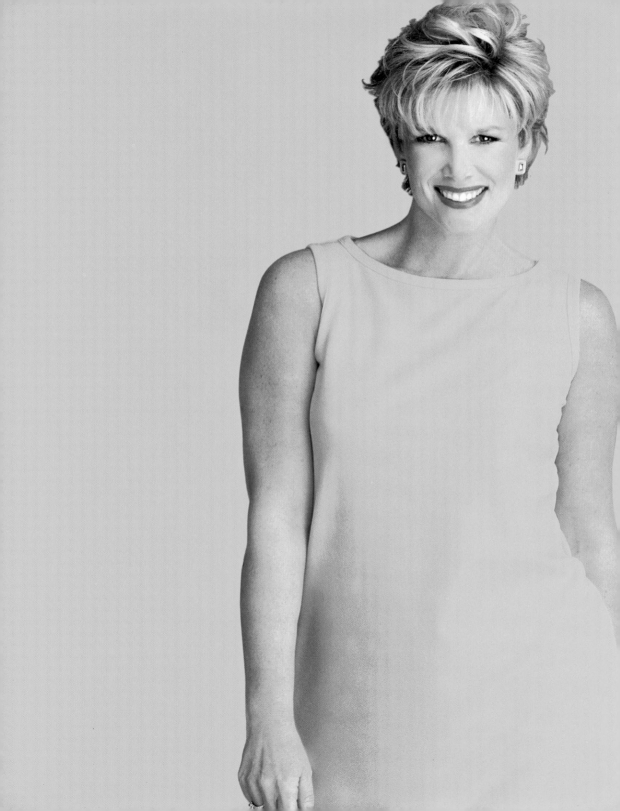

1 Living Healthier, Living Happier

My Incredible Journey

Life has been great these days. I have been on the most fantastic journey, seeking out great adventure for my mind, body, and spirit and reaching for a happier, healthier life. Over the past few years I have literally been transformed by fitness trainer Barbara Brandt and have finally regained control of my health. Barbara has been my cheerleader and my fitness conscience. It was because of her that I was finally able to take off and keep off those extra pounds that had been weighing down my life. She has taught me well, and I know that I will stay on this path of health and fitness.

You can make a decision to change your life at any time. Like most people facing the end-of-the-year crunch, I tend to get caught up in the hustle of the holiday season. That time of year gets filled with one obligation after another and enough stress to unhinge even a calm, well-balanced person. As 1995 drew to a close, for the first time ever I made a decision to take a week off just to relax and renew myself. I wanted to find a place where I could combine not only healthy eating and exercise but also lots of relaxation, yoga, positive thinking, and meditation. I wanted to keep an open mind and try lots of new things. I even thought I might like to try hiking. After asking around and doing some research, I headed off to the Golden Door Spa in San Diego, California.

I'd heard that each day at the "Door" started with a 4-mile hike up a mountain. My friends all thought I was crazy for wanting to wake up at 5:30 A.M. every day of my vacation! But the idea of climbing a mountain as the sun came up totally intrigued me.

It was still dark when our group of a dozen or so hikers gathered that first morning to share some herbal tea and fruit. After collecting our day packs, which held our mountaintop breakfast, we headed outside for our morning stretch.

Not long into the climb, I realized this was more than a pleasant walk and picnic. The group quickly divided into three smaller groups: a group of younger, more experienced hikers who seemed to bound up the mountain, a slower but steady middle group, and a third group who would lag behind with the thought of having to turn back a constant threat. "Oh, God! Please let me make it in to the middle group!" I quietly hoped to myself.

I learned a lot from that first morning climb. My heart was pounding so hard I could feel it in my ears. Breathing became more and more difficult. I was amazed that walking up a mountain was so hard for me. After all, I'd been working out regularly for over four years. Since I was in good shape I thought this hike would be a piece of cake. I didn't

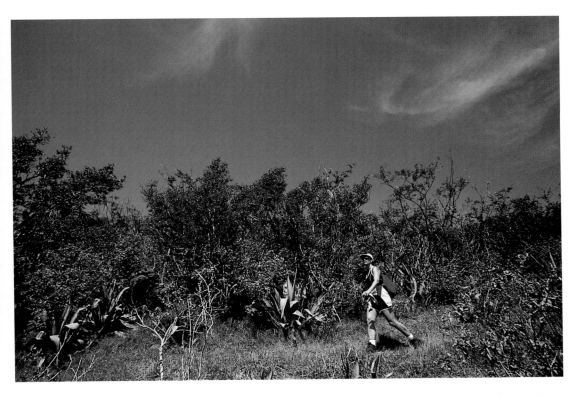

realize that different sports required specific training so I had a real eye-opener
finding myself in lowly group three.

In fact, there were many moments
when I almost gave in and turned back,
but to me, that was an unthinkable
choice. Our "shepherd" (I guess they're
called this because their job is to protect
us stray little lambs) would stop and let
me catch my breath and give me enough
encouragement to move me a little farther up the slope. About three quarters

*Be not afraid of going slowly; be afraid of
standing still.*

of the way to the top, just when I began
to believe I was really doing great, group
one came jogging past us—on their way
back *down*. I was so envious. But for now
my mission was to make it to the top of
this mountain and enjoy a well-deserved
breakfast.

To keep going, I envisioned myself on
the top of that mountain, overlooking

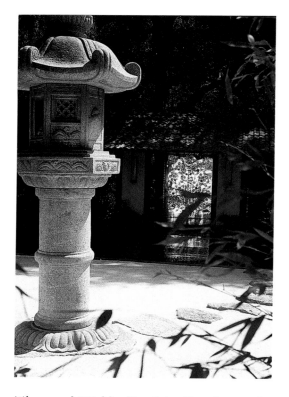

The actual "Golden Door" itself at the spa of the same name.

water. Not exactly a gourmet feast! But I did find a way to make the most of it: if you dip a bran muffin into yogurt, it's really not that bad. But just seeing the beautiful blue ocean all around and feeling the warmth of the sun on my face made that breakfast the best I'd ever had. Little did I know that the experience and accomplishment of reaching that mountaintop was about to set me off on a whole new journey in life.

I'd always wished I could be a healthy, nature-loving, spiritual, calm person who could indeed bound up a mountain if I so chose. And now here I was, actually taking that first step toward becoming the person I'd dreamed about.

The rest of our morning we kept busy with a Tai Chi morning stretch, funk aerobics, box aerobics, and strength training (my introduction to the world of weight lifting). Our efforts were rewarded with an afternoon of body scrubs, herbal wraps, massage, yoga, meditation training, and other relaxing treatments. In the evening we were invited into the kitchen for lessons on how to prepare healthy and delicious spa foods. This was clearly a favorite offering at the spa, and everyone joined in. At

the vast blue Pacific. In my mind's eye, I could really see myself up there. I don't know why, but that picture included me unpacking some kind of lavish breakfast spread. When I finally reached the top, I opened my pack and unwrapped my breakfast: a banana, an orange, a dry nonfat bran muffin, a small container of plain nonfat yogurt, and a bottle of

POTASSIUM BROTH

MAKES APPROXIMATELY 12 SERVINGS

This recipe is one of my favorites from the Golden Door. Take your leftover vegetables from the refrigerator and throw them into a pot. This drink is great to replace lost vitamins and minerals from a workout to help reduce lactic acid in the muscles after exercise.

46 ounces low-sodium
   vegetable juice
2 cups water
3 cups vegetable trimmings
   such as celery leaves,
   mushrooms, zucchini, onion,
   green onion, bell pepper,

parsley stems, lettuce,
   or carrots
1 teaspoon chili pepper
   flakes (optional)
1 teaspoon dry or
   1 tablespoon fresh basil

In a soup pot, combine the vegetable juice, water, vegetable trimmings, chili pepper flakes, and basil and bring the mixture to a boil. Reduce the heat and simmer about 40 minutes. Strain, discarding the solids. Serve the broth hot or cold.

NUTRITION *(per generous 1/2 cup serving):* CALORIES: 20; SATURATED FAT: 0G; TOTAL FAT: 0G (0% OF CALORIES); PROTEIN: 1 G (15% OF CALORIES); CARBOHYDRATES: 4 G (85% OF CALORIES); CHOLESTEROL: 0 MG; FIBER: 0 G; VITAMIN A: 783 IU; SODIUM: 26 MG; IRON: 1 MG; VITAMIN C: 24 MG

9:00 P.M. I fell into bed and experienced perhaps the rarest of all events for me: a full night's wonderful sleep.

The next day, the reporter in me stepped forward, and I started asking a lot of questions. I asked our guides for tips on how to make it up the trail more easily. I found I'd been expending too much energy taking steps that were too big. I was told to keep the movement below my waist, focusing on the butt and legs. The guides also gave me breathing techniques that kept my heart rate down and my spirits up.

Day two of climbing the mountain was still hard. But it was such a vast improvement over day one that I knew I had to go for day three. Next decision: would I sign that piece of paper at dinner opting for the 8-mile hike off the spa's campus—twice as long as today's? I found great consolation in knowing I wasn't the only one vacillating on whether to dare the bigger mountain range. But a new voice was speaking inside me now. It was not the old "what if this is too much for me…I don't know if I can do this" voice. This voice had an optimistic sound to it and made me

believe I could do anything. It was a loud and encouraging tone that broke through any assumptions I had regarding self-limits. "This is not too much for me…and I can do this!" bellowed from my heart and soul. I had made my choice: I would go for the 8 miles. I signed that piece of paper.

I approached day three with boundless confidence, though clearly this would be the most challenging climb of my stay. Only a handful of people decided to go that morning, and we derived great strength from each other. And, for added incentive, one of our guides let us in on the well-kept secret of this 8-mile climb: those who made it got to stop at Starbucks Coffee on the way back to the spa. Now, I know this may not sound like a big deal, but when you haven't had anything for four days but healthy spa cuisine, and no caffeine…it is!

As we approached the national park where we would do our hike, I was a bit nervous. I mean, c'mon, what was I thinking? I'd had trouble with the 4-mile climb; what made me think I could do 8 miles? What kind of masochist was I? Some women go to the Golden Door and never leave the place. They get

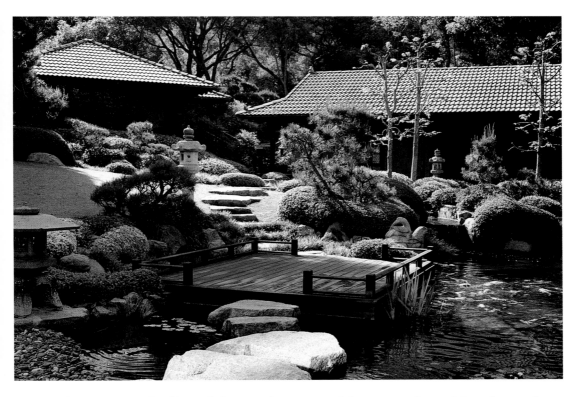

wrapped in seaweed, dipped in mud baths, and massaged with essential aromatic oils. They pamper themselves beyond belief...and I could be there with them. But noooooo, I had to climb this eight-mile mountain. Hello...anyone in there? Yes, a voice calling me to the top of the mountain. And it required an answer, one that could be found only at the peak.

As scared as I was by the thought of climbing a much more challenging dis-

One of the serene and peaceful gardens at the Golden Door.

tance, I actually found that hike easier and much more fun than the others. I also enjoyed the bond that formed between the few of us who had the courage to go that morning. The really cool thing was that nobody tried to show off. We all stayed together and supported each other's efforts. And yes, in the end, that coffee tasted like heaven.

I couldn't wait to get back to my room that night and share this incredible experience with my friends by phone. After talking with several close friends, I realized that the mountain climb was merely symbolic of what this whole trip encompassed for me. This was a journey of overcoming self-limits. I had never been willing to open myself up to so many new ideas and experiences: meditation, yoga, Tai Chi, and weight training. As my week progressed, I actually found myself inviting more new experiences and wondering how I could continue this journey in my "real life" back home. Only later would I realize its full impact. But the immediate effect of my stay at the Golden Door was that I returned to New York hell-bent on finding a way to build on my great new discoveries. Usually when people go to a spa, they have a great healthy week, vow they'll incorporate those experiences into life at home— and inevitably end up going back to their old ways. I was determined not to fall victim to inertia.

I was so determined, in fact, that from the airport in Los Angeles, I called my good friend (and, as you may recall, the co-author of this book) Laura Morton. My trainer, Barbara Brandt, was taking some time off to have her third daughter, and I was raring to go. I asked Laura to start researching gyms, to find a place where we could practice the muscle-building program introduced to me at the Door. (More on the importance of building muscle in Chapter 9.) Laura already had the answer to my question. How lucky can you get: the place she'd found, La Palestra, was directly across the street from the *Good Morning America* studio. So much for ever again using the "I just couldn't make it to the gym" excuse.

I was a bit reluctant at first to join La Palestra. I had read articles about their super-strict membership policy. I'd heard that if you didn't work out on a regular basis, for a minimum number of hours a week, they'd actually give you back your money and ask you to leave. How humiliating is that? (Many gyms are happy to take your money and never lay eyes on you again!) With my hectic schedule, I wasn't sure I could meet those minimum requirements. When I finally met with the staff, I heard another rule: if my goal was simply aes-

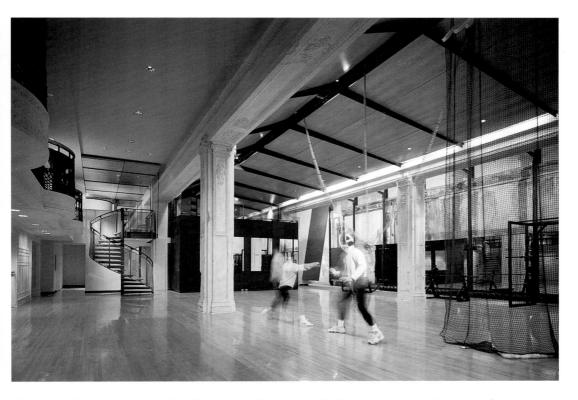

La Palestra—a masterpiece in architecture.

thetic, to lose ten pounds, they weren't interested in me as a member. *Huh?* It was explained to me that each member is an athlete in training, working to better his or her body, increase muscle mass, build endurance, tone muscles, and—lastly—to decrease body fat. That's why La Palestra calls itself a center for preventative medicine instead of a gym.

La Palestra epitomized everything I'd wanted to bring back from the spa: that philosophy of being good to yourself and taking care of your body. Wow, I was actually finding a way to fit those cool new teachings from the spa into my hectic New York life.

Most important, the staff eradicated from my thoughts forever the idea that "I have to go to the gym to lose weight." Let's face it, that's why people hate going to the gym in the first place. Pat Manocchia, the owner of La Palestra (and now our fitness expert on *GMA*), has a unique approach to fitness training. A former hockey player, he thinks like an athlete, and his goal is to make his clients think that way. Each member is tracked into a sport of his or her choice, with an individualized training program. Voilà! I was now an athlete in training! This made going to the gym exciting and fun, not a drag. Okay, great theory, but I still had one more thing to figure out: What sport was I training for, anyway? The New York City Marathon? Kayaking? Fencing? Boxing? (No, I don't think so.) Mountain climbing?

Whoa—stop right there! The memory of standing atop the southern California mountains, looking out into the blue Pacific Ocean, was still so vibrantly fresh in my mind that my choice was crystal clear: I would now be an athlete in training for a mountain climb. We set a date of June 5, 1996, to climb the Grand Tetons in Jackson Hole, Wyoming. That gave me six months to train. "Hey, I can do that," I told myself. And my usual partner in crime, Laura, agreed to join me.

Having a goal provided me with great inspiration every day. Pat started me on an interval walking-running program: walk a half mile, run a quarter mile, walk another half mile. I had never really been a runner before, mostly because I lacked endurance. I also had a problem with shin splints. (Take my advice on this one—buy yourself a good pair of running shoes. What a huge difference it's made for me.)

I learned that the way you build endurance is through a program that slowly increases your cardiovascular capacity. I worked my way through the half mile–quarter mile–half mile routine, on up to a half-mile run. What a high that was! And now I'm running three miles at a shot. If you had asked me a year ago if I'd ever be able to run any distance, I would have laughed at the thought. But then again, who would have believed I'd be training to climb the Grand Tetons?

Our training meant a rigorous schedule, working out for many hours each week. The winter of 1995 was a particularly snowy one in New York, and Pat used this opportunity to have us train as much as we could outside to experience walking in the snow. We had a record blizzard in January that year: some 24 inches fell in Manhattan. The entire city was closed down, which is quite rare for this metropolis. But there we were—Laura, Pat, me, and about a dozen other members of La Palestra—trudging through thigh-deep snow in Central Park. We walked all over the park for three hours. It was incredible to experience this in the middle of New York City. I had never realized there were so many hills in Central Park. By the time we stopped for our first food break, I was drenched with sweat (not perspiration, *sweat*). Pat brought pears for us to eat, along with sesame bars, which sort of resembled bird seed in their look and texture. The thrill of accomplishing this city hike inspired me to get serious about the rigorous training ahead.

The first few weeks I had to walk 10 miles on the treadmill at a 3-degree incline. By the third month (halfway there), I was walking 15 miles a week with the treadmill at a 9-degree incline. And in the last weeks before our trip, we added the experience of walking with our backpacks, filled with 20 to 30 pounds of weight, for 18 miles a week at a 12-degree incline. (That's like walking up a steep hill, rising 12 feet higher in the air for every 100 feet you walk.) In addition to that, we were supposed to log thirty minutes on the StairMaster at least three days a week *and* continue on our weight training program. I'm exhausted just thinking about it.

Just blocking out that much training time was tough, given my incredibly busy work schedule. In fact, as the date drew closer, I had some serious doubts about going through with the climb, because I'd started to fall behind in my training. Not for lack of desire, mind you, but because of my life filled with career commitments. The spring always means going on the road with *GMA*, and I was out of town for a couple of weeks. By the time things slowed down a little, there were only two weeks to go until I'd be looking up at those mountains.

Along with the physical training for this trip, I had to prepare for it mentally. As I always say, when the going gets tough, the tough go shopping, so...it was off to a real, heavy-duty mountain climbing store. The guys in that store showed—and, I might add, sold—me everything I needed to make this journey. I got down on the floor and tried out the sleeping bags. I stomped around

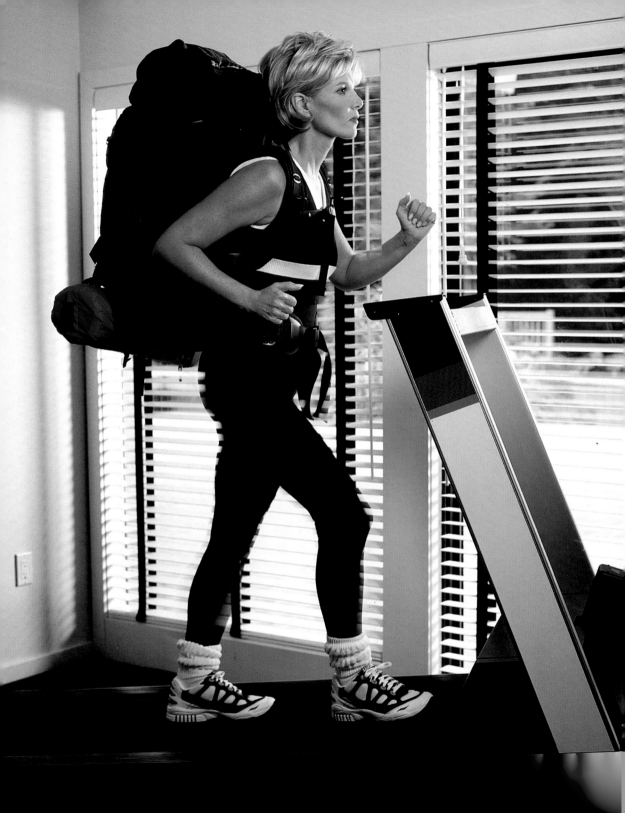

their rock field in my new hiking boots. I learned the difference among water resistant, water repellent, and waterproof. I bought snow pants, pile pants, a Gore-Tex jacket, and gloves. I bought glacier glasses, furry neck warmers, and thin sock liners. I even bought a headlamp with two extra batteries, and I picked out a great blue-and-gray backpack. Hey, these things were so expensive, I wanted it to say Gucci on it, you know what I mean? It was at that moment that I suddenly realized that the backpack I had just bought—with all of those other new goodies inside it—was the same backpack I was supposed to carry up a 13,000-foot mountain. Wait one cotton-picking minute. Is it too late to change my mind? How much do those extra batteries weigh, anyway?

I have never been known for my light packing skills, but no time like the present to hone that talent—and perfect it I did. In the end, my pack weighed as little as it possibly could for having as much in it as it did. Laura and I went to the drugstore the weekend before our

It's all uphill from here.

trip and bought mini-everythings: a tiny tube of toothpaste, a baby toothbrush, and even a mini-box of mini-pads. At least we had the advantage of being able to share a lot of our things.

The weekend prior to our departure, I invited Laura up to my home in Connecticut so that we could practice wearing our full packs. I live in a hilly community, so I thought it made sense to walk around my neighborhood for the practice—as if the little country town would somehow simulate the Teton Mountains. What was I thinking?

After donning our packs, now weighing in at 40 to 50 pounds, we made our way through my neighborhood. The first night we got a little overzealous. Though we left intending to go for a three-mile hike, we managed to walk six miles. We found ourselves, post-dusk, still a good mile or so from home. But like good Girl Scouts, we'd left home prepared. I put on my headlamp and lit our path back home.

Backpackers are not the most common sight in my Connecticut town, so people were looking at us twice from every passing car. If only they had known it was me under all that gear! As we approached my house, standing there in my driveway were my children and my good friend Scot Evans. They were moments away from getting into the car and heading out to search for us. They roared with laughter at the sight of Laura and me coming up the driveway in full gear, headlamps and all. I must admit we were quite a sight!

With only a few days remaining before leaving for Jackson Hole, my nerves were growing shakier by the moment. I kept asking myself if I could really do this. When I started training, I'd announced on *Good Morning America* that I was preparing for a mountain climb. Originally I said I was training for Mount Kilimanjaro, which is still a goal of mine. Many viewers sent me information about their own climbs.

A few nights before our climb, Laura and I watched a video sent to me by a woman named Doris Quinn. It was a firsthand account of her trip to Africa and her climb up Kilimanjaro. We sat and listened to this gentle, soft-spoken woman slowly reveal the most intimate moments of her trip, shown to us through the magic of videotape. Doris is in her mid-fifties, and here she was

climbing the tallest mountain in Africa! We witnessed her self-doubt as she approached the summit, nearly 20,000 feet in the air. She convinced herself to go on when she hardly had another breath left. Her determination to reach that summit became an inspiration to me in those days before my trip. "If Doris can do it, then I'll be damned, so can I!" When Doris reached the peak, she was so overjoyed she cried uncontrollably. As we saw Doris make her dream come true, Laura and I wept along with her. (Okay, so we're both a couple of weenies.) We knew then that the days that lay ahead were bound to change our lives forever. It was at that moment that we made a pact between us to be very open about how we were feeling on our climb. Neither one of us needed to be a hero on this trip. I'd also received several articles on the perils of altitude sickness, which prompted us to talk about the possibility of getting sick on the mountain. Just to be secure, I called my doctor and got a prescription for Diamox, a medicine commonly used to combat altitude sickness. As you will see, it was one of the most important items I packed.

Ready or not, on June 5, 1996, we

were on our way to the airport, headed to Jackson Hole, Wyoming. Pat is big on the team-playing theory, so our group had met at La Palestra on that warm, early summer day to travel together. It's a long trip from New York to Wyoming, and a two-hour time difference. I'd started my day at 4:00 A.M. to host *GMA*, and by the time we arrived at our motel in Jackson Hole, I was completely wiped out. We checked in, grabbed a quick bite to eat, and hit the hay, as they say out west. I knew that this would be my best chance for a good night's sleep for the next few days, so I relished every moment.

We awoke at 6:00 A.M. and made our final preparations to leave for the mountain. It was a magnificent morning. The sun was rising over the snow-capped peaks, and the wet grass looked green and lush. Here we were, ready to go, fifteen climbers, four guides, fifteen backpacks, helmets, ice axes, snow-climbing boots, and crampons. (No, a crampon is not something women use once a month. It's a device that attaches to the bottom of your boots to give you a better grip on a snow-slick mountain. It looks kind of like a bear's claw.)

Wait, where am I supposed to put all of this extra equipment? I asked myself. Just when I thought my pack couldn't get any heavier, they added another ten pounds. Jim Williams, the guide assigned to watch over Laura and me, helped us secure the equipment and make our final adjustments. We were able to leave our everyday clothes at the motel for our return on Saturday. Laura grabbed our suitcases and headed to the van that would shuttle us to the foot of the mountain. As luck would have it, she pulled a muscle in her back picking up a heavy bag. It really knocked the wind out of her, and I could tell that she was in a lot of pain.

We boarded the van. Toni McGinley, a physical therapist from the gym, worked on Laura's back. We drove five minutes out of downtown Jackson Hole, and there they were: the Grand Tetons. They were a lot *bigger* than I thought they would be and incredibly imposing. Suddenly I felt small and frail. The peaks were almost completely covered in snow, and the sun reflected the most extraordinary glare back at us.

Was I the *only* one starting to feel scared and nervous?

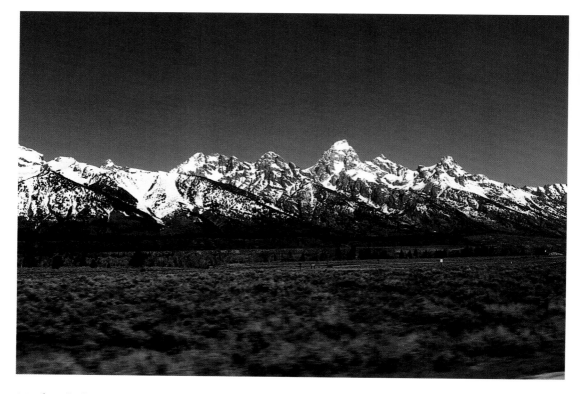

My first look at the Tetons.

Earlier that morning, Pat had had us fill out a psychological profile on how we were feeling. Was it too late to change my answers?

The scenery was breathtaking. I use that word purposefully because my breath and my ability to breathe were very much on my mind. I have had mild bouts of asthma over the years, and I feared that the altitude might trigger it. I had come prepared with inhalers, but still, that worry weighed heavy on my mind. A million other questions, doubts, and fears ran through my head. Am I strong enough to do this? Should I be wearing a T-shirt instead of a turtleneck? Will I be too hot from climbing or too cold because there is so much snow?

I kept thinking about my daughter Jamie's equestrian trainer, Kip Rosenthal. When she knows that one of the horses

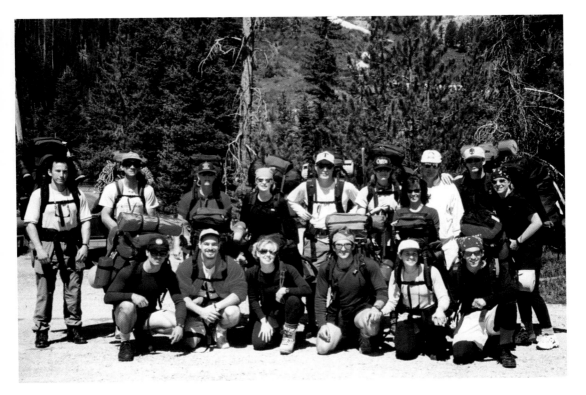

might balk at the idea of going over a certain jump, Kip always tells Jamie to be confident, positive, and aggressive. She says, "You have to want to go over a jump more than the horse *doesn't* want to go over. The horse derives its confidence from you." Well, I had to want to get to the top of that mountain more intensely than I feared that I couldn't do it.

Laura turned around and looked at me and didn't say anything for a minute. I thought she was going to say that she

Our La Palestra climbing group ready for our climb: (top) John Descarfino, Tom Turiano, me, Holly Perkins, Steve Knutson, Jackie Adams, Steve Potter, John Aslop, Laura Morton; (bottom) Mark Tenore, Dan Thomas, Nora Brennan, Pat Manocchia, Deborah Wasserman, Tony Moody.

couldn't go through with the climb, that she was in too much pain. I was preparing myself for her not going, which really scared me, because we'd

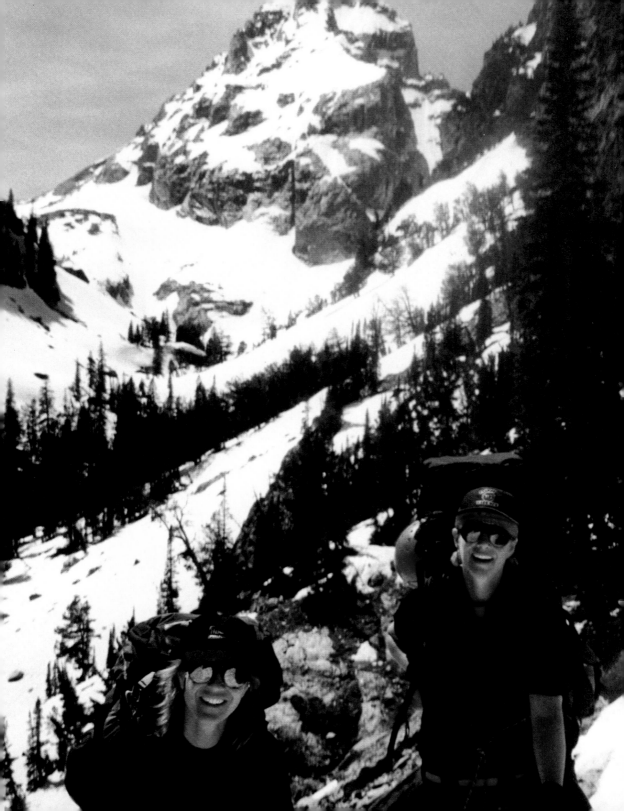

been deriving such strength and courage from each other. After a long pause, she just smiled and said, "*This* is going to be really cool!"

As we pulled onto the road leading to the entrance to the park, a helicopter hovered overhead, practicing picking up stretchers from the ground. They were training for emergency rescues. This was *not* what I wanted to see just before my trip!

Looking up at the beautiful mountain, we could see an incredible, magical waterfall coming from melting snow. Just above that point, I saw what at first glance appeared to be skiers' tracks.

Jim Williams, our guide, explained that those were actually fresh avalanche chutes and tracks. Oh, great! Our guides also warned us against keeping food in our tents, because of marmots and bears. A marmot looks a little like a beaver crossed with a raccoon. Apparently, if they smell food, they will come into your tent to find it. I'm sure our guides felt obligated to prepare us for the worst, but

Underneath our silly smiles we're actually thinking, "Are we really going to climb to the top of that?"

since there's a lot of wildlife up in the mountains, I was not taking any chances.

I had imagined the hike to base camp would be fairly easy. We were only going from 6,000 to 8,200 feet, and the estimate was only around four hours. Well, it turned out to be one hell of a climb. Within the first hour we had to change into hard-shell hiking boots and gaiters to protect us from the snow. Gaiters are shell-like covers that you wrap around your calves to keep snow from getting in your boots.

It was hot, and the grade was amazingly steep right from the start. I worried about my endurance, my breathing, and my heart rate, which was racing. Most of the La Palestra climbers were in their twenties and thirties, and here I was taking up this sport at forty-five! It was hard for me to keep up, but I was thinking positively, determined just to do the best that I could. If the climb to base camp was this tough, though, how would I do on our actual summit climb?

After a while, the scenery took my mind off my fear. Laura and I stopped a lot to use our camera and video recorder. I was overwhelmed by nature's beauty. Below me was a small lake that was the

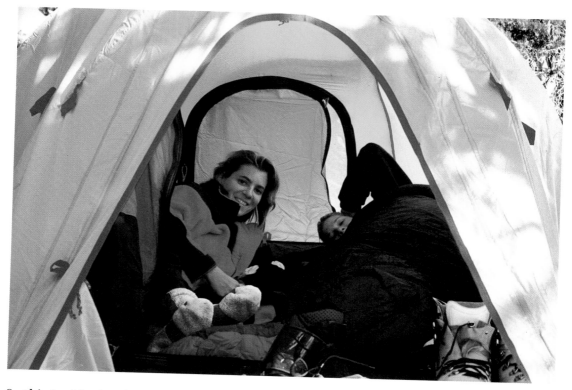

*So **this** is altitude sickness!*

deepest blue I had ever seen. The path we were taking was narrow and snow-covered. The snow softened in the heat of the day, becoming almost slushy. We walked through streams and under waterfalls. I couldn't believe I was there, doing what I was doing. I was using walking sticks, which are like adjustable ski poles, to help me keep my balance. We made it to our second resting point,

where our guides implored us to drink water. They explained that it is especially important to keep hydrated in the mountains and that we were losing more water than usual because of the climbing and the sweating.

The last bit of our day's hike was incredibly steep and difficult. I was beginning to feel dizzy and nauseated. I could see the field of tents set up at base camp in the distance, and I just wanted to be there so badly. Laura and I reached base camp around 5:30 P.M. Most of the group was already there and unpacked. Okay, so we took our time getting there —but we got there, right? We made it.

I was so incredibly tired that I couldn't get my sleeping bag rolled out fast enough to lie down inside our tent. I couldn't even tell if the slope I was resting on went up or down. My head was now pounding, and I found it impossible to get up to do anything. Surely this feeling couldn't get any worse. But it did, and I realized I had been struck with altitude sickness. Thank goodness that we'd seen Doris's tape before we left, and taken her advice to bring some Diamox. I took half a pill and tried to get some sleep while the others bustled about and prepared for dinner. I couldn't move. I felt awful. I just wanted to stay lying down, but our guide, Jim, convinced me that moving around and drinking lots of water would actually make me feel better. I was feeling especially dehydrated, so I drank a lot. One thing they forgot to tell me about Diamox is that it's also a diuretic, so the more I drank...do I have to explain? Under normal circumstances, this would be a welcome side effect for me. However, with the way I was feeling,

the 20-degree temperature, and—oh, yes —the fact that I was on the side of a mountain with no official plumbing, this prospect was not quite as appealing.

Well, I did get up and move around a bit that night, but the thought of food disgusted me. Laura practically force-fed me a few spoonfuls of chicken noodle soup (and managed to get the recipe from our guide at the same time). Nothing appealed to me at the time but the thought of getting back to my tent. I suffer such sleep deprivation and fatigue as it is, I knew that I would need every ounce of strength to go on. I took another half of a Diamox before bed and hoped that tomorrow would be a better day.

It was Friday. We woke up around 7:30, and I thought I was feeling better. In fact, I thought I was up for a hearty breakfast. I started to get dressed, and again felt completely exhausted. It was work just to put on those heavy hiking boots, but somehow I managed. I headed on down to the breakfast area. Uh-oh! Nothing looked good to me. One of the guides poured hot water over a bowl of granola and strawberries. It was palatable, but I can't say that I was really into the mountain food. Today would be a

GRAND TETON CHICKEN NOODLE SOUP

SERVES 10

This recipe is from one of our climbing guides, Tom Turiano. It's a simple delicious recipe for the best medicine anyone could need...even on a mountaintop! If you're making this at home, you can use tap water, which doesn't need to be treated beforehand.

2 ½ quarts bottled water or stream
    water treated with iodine tablets
    to prevent contamination
2 chicken bouillon cubes
1 pound whole wheat or spinach
    rotelli noodles

½ cup dried vegetable flakes
1 cup potato flakes
2 cans white meat chicken
Garlic powder to taste
Italian herbs to taste
Parmesan cheese (optional)

Bring the water and bouillon cubes to a boil in a large soup pot. Add the noodles, vegetable flakes, and potato flakes and cook until the noodles are almost done but still firm. Stir in the chicken, garlic powder, and Italian herbs and heat through. Add cheese to taste, if desired.

practice day to better prepare us for our big climb. We would learn how to use those crampons, tie in to the ropes, and to perform what's called self-arrest. As I started to get moving, I felt much more human. Laura and I headed up the mountain to hone our skills for tomorrow. They made us put on our snow pants and jackets—even though it was quite warm—because we were going to practice falling down. You slide easier in the nylon-type fabrics; you also slide faster, for what that's worth. The guides went over the basics of self-arrest. This is a helpful technique to stop yourself from falling down a mountain. Basically, you plunge your ice ax into the snow as you fall, and assume a position that secures you. We practiced three different ways. First, we slid out on our tushes and rolled over, plunged our axes into the snow, and went into what's called the cat position, like a kitty cat arching its back. The second time, we slid face forward on our stomachs and had to do the same thing —but also turn ourselves around so that we ended up facing uphill. Finally, we tried it sliding backward on our backs down the mountain, and again had to finish on our hands and knees, facing uphill. Self-arrest means stopping your fall on a 45-degree slope with an ice ax. This is a dangerous tool, and you must be very careful how you hold it. I perfected this skill pretty quickly, because I soon realized that the farther I allowed myself to fall, the farther I'd have to walk back up that mountain to try it again!

We enjoyed a mountainside lunch of French bread, Brie, sprouts, cucumbers, and grapes. It was a spectacular day! In the late afternoon we headed down the mountain to base camp to rest for tomorrow's early morning climb. Just how early? We were told that we would be awakened at 1:30 A.M.—that's awfully early, even for me! I took a Diamox before I retired and again drank lots of water. I think that everyone—including me—was asleep by 8:00 P.M. After all that work, it wasn't too hard.

It seemed like only a minute had gone by, but suddenly it was 1:30 in the morning. The time had come. All we had trained for, all the hours of sweat and determination, boiled down to the next few hours. It was an unusually warm morning—or middle of the night, anyway. The chinook winds were blowing a warm and eerie breeze. All of us were quiet and nervous as we quickly pulled ourselves together into four groups. In the darkness of the night, guided only by the tracks of the person in front and by the dim light of the moon, we were on our way.

The faster, more experienced climbers quickly pulled ahead of the rest. By the end of first half hour, all I could see was the distant glow of their headlamps. Laura and I were once again bringing up the rear. We decided to go at our own pace and to go only as far as we could take ourselves. The sound of my heartbeat was as loud in my head as an African tribal drum. The rhythm set the pace for my steps. Every step was slow and calculated. I wanted to expend as little energy as I

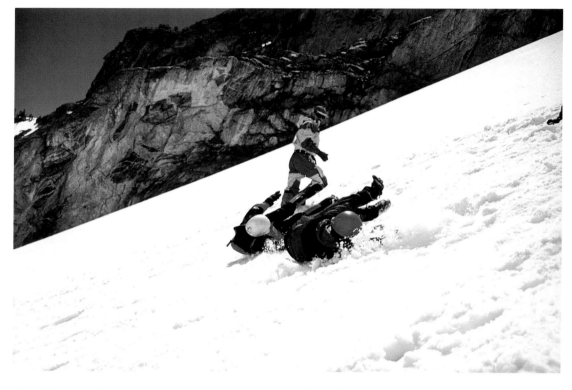

I've fallen, and I can't get up!

could, to keep myself going. To say that this wasn't a dramatic experience is like calling childbirth pain-free. The most interesting thing about making the early part of this hike in the dark was that I couldn't really see what I was climbing. It was kind of like painting the windows of an airplane black if you are afraid to fly. What you can't see can't scare you.

Just as I found my confidence for the

first time that morning, the wind kicked up and it started to rain. It seemed surreal. Me, climbing a mountain in the middle of the night, knee deep in snow, in the rain! I couldn't have made this story up if I tried, mostly because I could never have imagined *me* as the main character!

Fortunately the rain soon stopped and the sun peeked over the horizon behind us, signaling another beautiful morning about to break. Laura stopped, pulled out

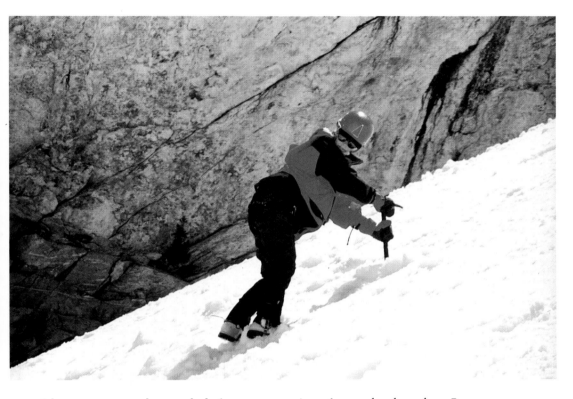

our video camera, and recorded the sunrise. We wanted to capture this moment forever. We reached a relatively flat part of the mountain and now confronted something they never prepared us for in our training—and it was the one thing that really freaked Laura out. This flat land was a huge mass of rocks and boulders that we had to navigate like soldiers walking through a mine field. And we had to do it in heavy hiking boots (something like ski boots), while carrying huge backpacks. Laura was very unsure of her balance, and as it turned out, a lot of climbers had trouble making their way through this seemingly harmless yet incredibly intimidating place. We stopped and sat on a huge rock to allow Laura to regain her poise.

Not far beyond that point, Jim suggested we review our options. If we chose to continue up this path, we couldn't "summit" with everyone else because we were running out of daylight hours. But,

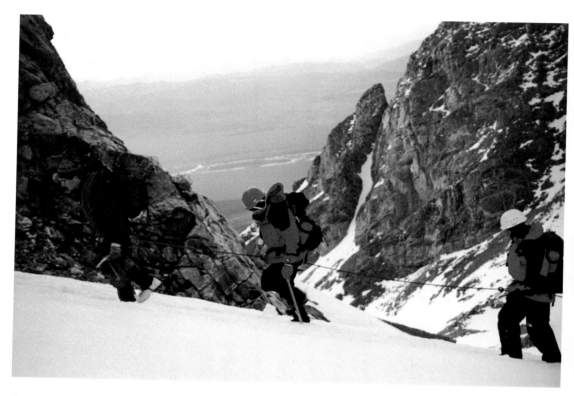

Forging ahead.

as he pointed out, there are many different summits, and just because you don't climb the tallest one doesn't make it any less of an achievement. Our goal wasn't necessarily to get to the very top of the mountain that morning; we just wanted to take ourselves beyond anywhere we'd ever been. So we agreed to change our course. We would summit the 11,650-foot saddle of the Tetons instead.

As we made our way toward our personal summit, Steve Knutson, a fellow climber from La Palestra, joined us. He too had realized that this mountain was a lot tougher than he had anticipated. I was so glad we were there for him and he was there for us. Together we experienced something quite different from the rest of the group but in some ways much the same. No, I decided, I would not be disappointed with this summit. It was grand and glorious, and it was an

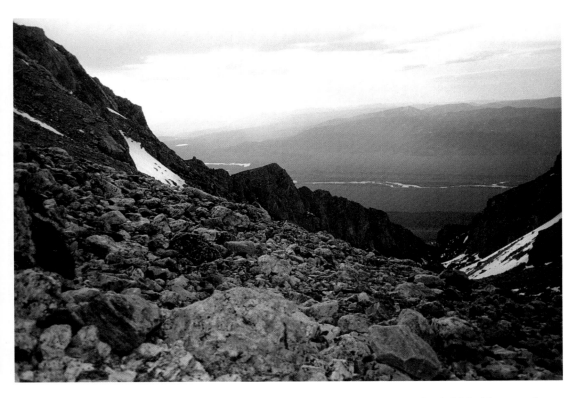

accomplishment way beyond my wildest dreams.

As we approached our summit, I could see forever. Idaho to my right, Montana to my left—and there I was, standing on top of the world in Wyoming. It was so cool! That moment made all of the sickness and exhaustion completely worthwhile. My heart raced with joy and excitement at what I was seeing, what I was feeling, and how far I had come. Those African drums in my

The treacherous boulder field halfway to the top of the Tetons.

head had gone away, and I was hearing instead the sounds of vastness. I was so proud of myself: proud that I had broken out of self-doubt and continued against the odds, proud that I could share this experience with friends, proud that I had gone beyond my own threshold. No more self-limits—that would be my new philosophy.

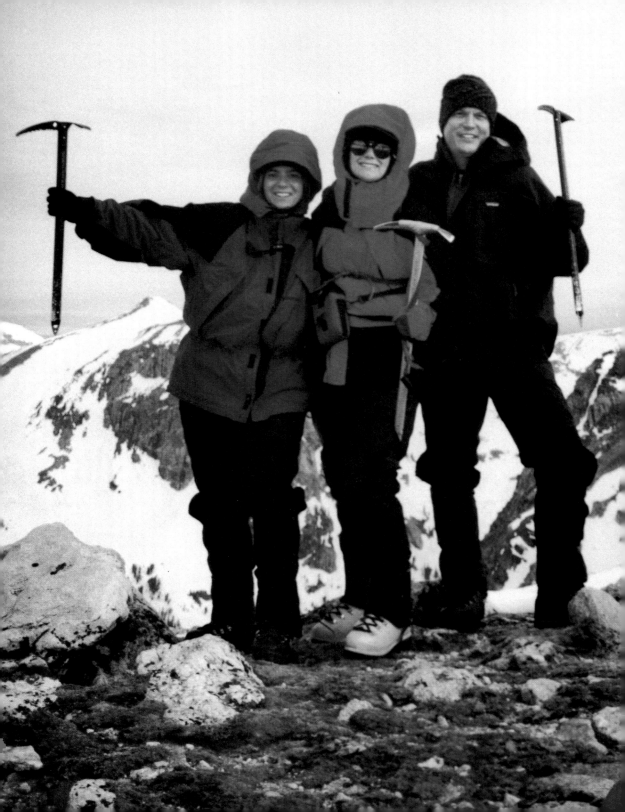

Reaching the summit that morning represented a lot more to me than the physical accomplishment. I knew that from now on, because of that experience, I would view many things in life differently. You see, we have choices about the way our lives will be. On that mountain, I could have caved in to all of the challenges. The old me would not have gone through with this journey. Oh, I would have had the desire, but not necessarily the will to follow through. And just as I decided to change my course that morning and continue toward my goal, so can you change the course of your life. It all starts with a simple choice. If you are unhappy or unhealthy, it is your choice to make a change and do something about it. If you continue to live your life the same way, even though you're unhappy, unexcited, and overwhelmed, no one can help you change it. Something's got to give! And that's you. You've got to give yourself a better life. There's no reason to resign yourself to a life that's not fulfilling. So go for it. It's your choice.

We did it! Laura, Steve Knutson, and me at our own personal summit.

We Choose What We Will Become

It's no secret that I chose to make a life change at age thirty-nine. I was fifty pounds overweight, unhappy with my life, and downright frightened about my health. It took a lot of attempts and failures before I figured out a way to succeed. And there's no magic bullet. It takes time, effort, desire, *and* the right information and strategy to make that change. One thing I knew for sure, in the deepest part of my soul, was that if I got healthy, I would get happy. So I changed the way I ate, and I changed the way I thought about and perceived food and exercise. Once I became aware of my inner power, I became the captain of my ship, so to speak, and I needed to plot a new course to discover this buried treasure...*me!*

Other public people have gone on this inner search. One of the most remarkable transformations was that of talk show host Ricki Lake. Ricki always wanted to be in show business: she'd pursued it since she was a young child. At age nineteen, she landed the leading role in the cult film *Hairspray.* Within a

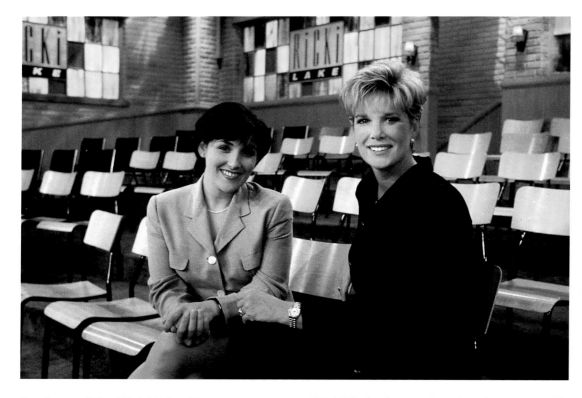

On the set of The Ricki Lake Show.

year, Ricki hit it big again, with a recurring role in the Emmy-winning TV show *China Beach*. But *China Beach* was canceled soon after, and at twenty-one, Ricki found herself single, unemployed, scrambling to make her rent, and weighing over 250 pounds. She dedicated the next three years to reinventing herself and losing over 100 pounds.

Having started over in 1993, the *new*

Ricki Lake began hosting her own talk show and is now one of today's most successful daytime talk show hosts. Ricki represents to me a woman who really understands what it means to take control of your health and happiness. She clearly understood that she did have a choice.

I interviewed Ricki on the set of her show in 1995 for my ABC-TV prime-time special *Behind Closed Doors,* where she revealed what she felt was her biggest accomplishment. I think she surprised a lot of people with her description of her proudest feat:

After you lose over one hundred pounds, I was shouting to the world—to anyone who would listen to me... because it's my biggest accomplishment. You know, it's something that I never ever thought that I would be able to do. And compared to having a talk show, this is what's really hard...losing weight and keeping it off. So you know, at the same time, I'm actually tired of talking about it, because I have been at the same weight for a long time now, it's just that I'm still thrilled to death about it.

Probably the most visible person Americans have watched in their search for healthy, happy role models is fellow talk show host Oprah Winfrey. She has talked often about being at a high of 237 pounds and at a low of 142 pounds. She says she tried every food fad known and every diet of the moment, but she would only gain back the weight she'd lost and wind up feeling guilty and weak. She explained:

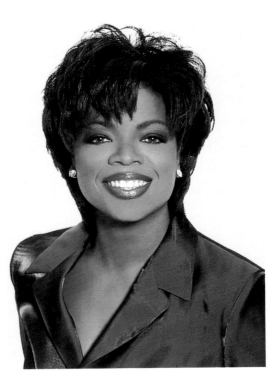

Oprah Winfrey—a true inspiration.

Having tried a gajillion diets, I understand how when we want to lose weight, we tend to look for the answer outside ourselves. We want a magic solution—a secret formula. I used to wish somebody would just tell me the answer—show me ways. Someone did. But I've also learned what Glinda, the Good Witch told Dorothy in The Wizard of Oz: *"You always had it.*

You always had the power." The real secret is within you.

After four years of searching for and finally finding the right fitness philosophy, her trainer, Bob Greene, says she's a different person who is satisfied with herself. Oprah says that she has become a happier person who can handle stress just fine.

Needless to say Oprah, Ricki, and I are not alone in this struggle. A recent *Shape* magazine article states that 50 million Americans are battling the bulge. They are frightened for their health and seeking happier, fuller lives. How did we get here, with so many people at a crisis point? Well, partly because of the barrage of health messages, we're "getting it" now, understanding that we need healthy bodies and healthy minds for a quality life. In addition, more people in this country are over the age of fifty than ever before.

The first of 76 million baby boomers, born between 1946 and 1964, are turning fifty this year, so happy birthday to the fastest-growing segment of our population. Let's celebrate by giving ourselves the gift of a happier, healthier next fifty

years. According to Dr. James Rippe, "those who live physically active lives will not only lower their risk of chronic disease but also enhance their daily functional capacity and, in general, lead happier, fuller, more energetic lives."

When you factor in the powerful benefits of physical activity on heart disease, cancer, diabetes, and weight control along with other known benefits, such as improved mental health and reduced risk of osteoporosis, it is easy to see why it has been estimated that inactivity results in 250,000 needless deaths a year. Our poor habits are actually killing us. Committing to a simple lifestyle change, choosing to eat mindfully, and participating in regular physical activity will help keep your mind and body healthier and can actually slow the functional decline of aging. According to a recent Yankelovich survey, one of the primary reasons for adult inactivity is not knowing where to begin. This book will strip away that old excuse by helping you to understand that health and activity go together, no matter what your age or starting fitness level.

Some people think they are too old to start all this running around. But the older we get, the more important it becomes to exercise. Our bones lose density and our muscles actually shrink! All that sitting around is like playing a foolish game of Russian roulette with our hearts. Simple tasks that we take for granted, like getting out of a chair or walking, will become increasingly difficult as we age if we don't exercise regularly.

You may already be actively participating in life. You do aerobics, go for a jog or a walk, play tennis, or even mountain-climb. You may have discovered, as I did, that physical activity not only brings this host of body benefits but also makes you feel good about yourself and enlivens the spirit. It keeps you feeling younger and more energetic. By knowing your needs and seeing that each one is met, you help choose what you'll become in later years. It's *your* future, and it's *your* choice. I want to help you blaze your own trail to a fit mind and body, and be there to support your efforts.

Finding the Perfect Balance

My life, like most people's, is full of roles, or layers. I'm a mother, a daughter, a friend. I have a career. I'm single—but dating. I balance my day by getting up before the sun, and while I find time to fulfill my many commitments to others, I now make sure to find time for my own needs as well. It has become a priority for me to find that balance in my life. I have figured out that I will survive life's ups and downs and that I can't look to anyone else for my personal happiness.

Have you ever driven a car, maybe listening to the radio, and suddenly you realize you've arrived where you were going, yet can't recollect the trip? You couldn't describe any landmarks you passed or how long the trip took. You were too distracted to notice. Well, I'm here to tell you that your life is like that car ride. Don't miss the ride. The journey is just as important as the destination.

While on vacation last summer, I was lying on a chaise longue relaxing and taking in a little sun, and I was struck by a particular song playing on the stereo. It was Barbra Streisand singing "On a Clear Day." Funny, I had heard that song a thousand times before and even sung along a time or two. (Don't we all sing along with Barbra, wishing our voices were as good as hers?) Anyway, I guess I had never been so receptive to the meaning of that song, which really asks you to look around you and see who you are. It stresses living in the moment, and that life is not about where you're going but about where you are, in the here and now. I'll be the first to admit that I have lived my life on such a fast track that I haven't always stopped to enjoy each moment along the way, and I have probably missed some good ones. But now that I have a clearer vision, I don't miss them anymore.

It is necessary to find a balance in your life so that you can clarify your vision and appreciate all of life's moments. Balance is defined as a stable state. It stands to reason that if you put too much focus on one area of your life (say, work), then another area (like family) will suffer. Your life becomes unbalanced.

Think about it for a moment. You are consumed with finishing a presentation for work, under the pressure of a deadline. Inevitably your focus is primarily on that project. After all, you don't want to risk losing your job, right? But at what cost? You neglect your home, your family, and worst of all yourself. You don't eat properly, you're not sleep-ing enough—generally speaking, you aren't taking care of yourself or your health. Does that seem like a fair trade-off to you? I know that my body reacts to this kind of situation by just shutting down. Every time I feel pulled in twenty different directions, I eventually get sick. I get a sore throat, a cough, and my energy level drops through the floor. That doesn't seem very productive, does it? Once I get sick, my job suffers, and I get caught up in that horrible cycle. I am out of balance.

"Women are always being tested . . . but ultimately, each of us has to define who we are individually and then do the very best job we can to grow into that."

HILLARY RODHAM CLINTON

Balance in your life means coordinating your physical well-being with your mental well-being. It's also the connection between your heart and your head. Balance may sometimes require courage

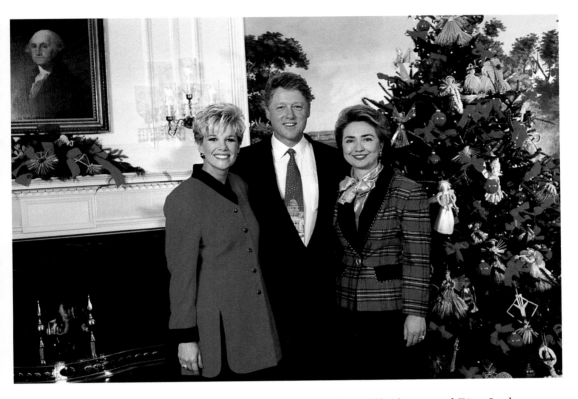

to try new things that may or may not work out for you.

I have definitely noticed an attitude shift in my circle of friends. It suggests that we all want something more out of life than we did in the past. I can't open up a magazine these days without reading about some "spiritual awakening," the benefits of meditation, or a stream of new findings on exercise and nutrition. I

President Bill Clinton and First Lady Hillary Rodham Clinton greeting me at a White House Christmas party.

think these articles reflect our search for something more than just achieving physical health, a great career, or even having a family. The direction seems to be finding a balance of all the things that make up our lives.

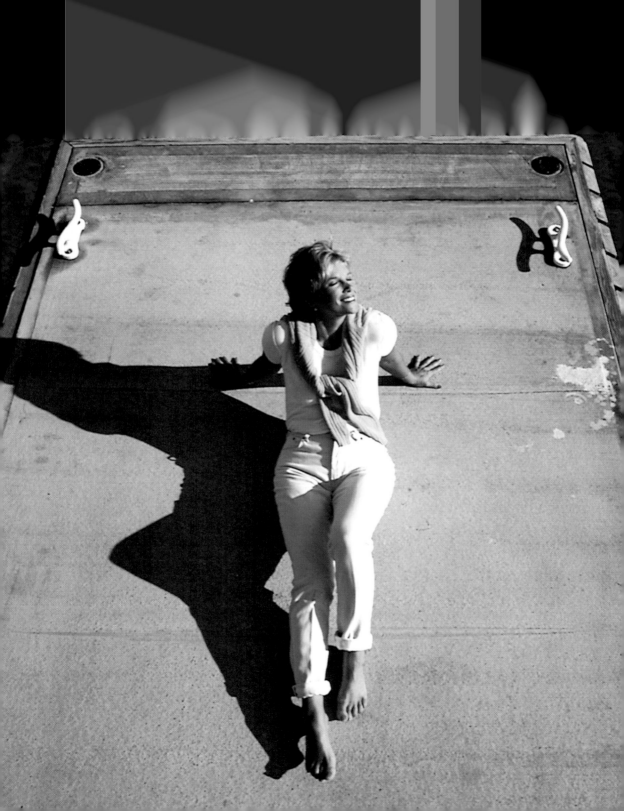

2 Don't Wait for Good Things to Happen

*Know the true value of time; snatch, seize, and enjoy
every moment of it.*

—LORD CHESTERFIELD

W hy is it that some people are able to take very
little information and seem to turn their lives
around instantly, while others, equipped with
exactly the same information, can't seem to make
anything work? The answer is actually pretty simple. Those who do, don't just take the information
—they take action. What sets apart the winners of
this world is that they put their thoughts into
action instead of passively waiting around for things
to change. These are the people who are living their

dreams instead of sitting around trying to figure out the best way to go, or waiting to "get in the mood." It's that old law of inertia: We have to move in order to achieve movement in our lives.

I think I have always known that you can't just wait for good things to happen, and that might have a good deal to do with why I am where I am today. I recently started thinking about fresh things I could do to add more movement in my life. I wanted to challenge myself creatively by using my skills and experience as a television host in new ways. I was recently asked by a well-known sitcom producer if I had ever considered doing my own sitcom. I laughed and explained to him that even though I had spent my whole career in show business, I really didn't consider myself an actress. His response took me aback: he not only disagreed but went on and on about how what I do every day hosting a live two-hour television show makes me one of the best actresses on the tube! "You can't possibly be enchanted by every single guest I have watched you interview for the last twenty years," he said, "but you make the viewer believe that you are. If that's not acting, I don't know what is."

Well, I don't agree with him completely; I *do* enjoy those interviews, but acting is not one of the skills I would put on my résumé. It *was* a lot of fun doing guest appearances on *Murphy Brown,* but as long as I am confessing, I'll also tell you that I was unbelievably nervous and absolutely sure that I would forget my lines. After twenty-three years in front of the camera! (Guess I hadn't perfected my positive thinking skills yet.)

While I have had cameos in *Free Willy 2* and *What About Bob?* and have loved the challenge of producing my specials, I've always had a secret wish, one I never expressed to anyone—not my co-workers, my bosses, or even my friends. I'm not even sure where this desire came from, but it kept returning over the years: I wanted to direct. I figured I must know *something* about it—after all, I'd been sitting on the other side of the camera all those years. I knew what cuts, pans, and dissolves were, and I understood lighting. But if you didn't study directing in school, how do you convince someone that you can do it?

Just like a young film school student, I figured that I would have to start out on my own, with a modest budget. I would have to make my own version of a home movie. But being the pragmatic person that I am, I needed a valid subject for the film. So I came up with my grand idea: I would give my then twelve-year-old daughter Lindsay a chance to gain professional experience as a dancer in a music video. Lindsay had been a Ford model (the agency, not the car company) for a year and had passionately studied dance since age ten. She had tons of raw talent, but really needed some professional experience. So I decided to produce and direct my first music video, MTV-style. In order to pull this task off, I had to swallow my pride and call in some favors. And, boy, did I ever. I went to every corner of my industry…all right, so I hit up all of my friends, but that's what a good producer does! I called upon Laura, who's a television producer when she's not co-writing books with me, to help me pull the crew and location together. And I called my dear friend, a former director of *GMA*, Bob McKinnon, to guide me through the directing process for the first time. We shot on a Brooklyn soundstage, which we redesigned to look like an artist's loft, complete with graffiti, exposed brick walls, and even a motorcycle. We filled

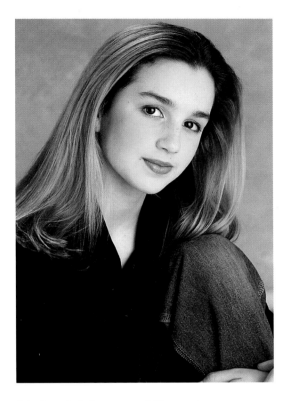

Lindsay Leigh on a modeling assignment.

this funky set with smoke, added really cool stage lighting, and hired professional backup dancers straight from the stages of Broadway! We went for the works and we all had a blast. For Lindsay it was fun to have this chance to be a star.

For me it was an adventure. I gave myself the opportunity to do something that I might not otherwise have been able to do, and then I took the ball and

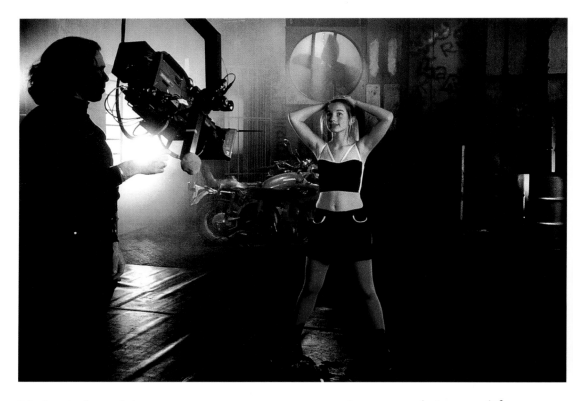

Lindsay in front of the cameras.

ran with it. I didn't wait for Francis Ford Coppola to call me to direct his next great film. (That could have been a pretty long wait!)

I was extremely lucky to have the ability to tap into the many contacts I had made through the years to pursue my dream, but the truth is we all have resources, friends, and opportunities we haven't even tapped yet. If you take a proactive approach in your life, you too can make good things happen. It really has nothing to do with who you are but rather with how you tackle something. You have to take action, approach it with a positive attitude, and have the desire to grow personally. That's the secret to making good things happen. Theodore Roosevelt said it like this: "Whenever you are asked if you can do a job, tell 'em, 'Certainly I can!'—and get busy and find out how to do it."

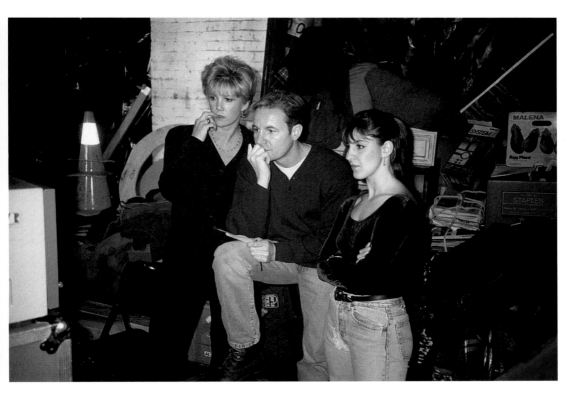

Just Do It!

"Even if you're on the right track, you'll get run over if you just sit there."

WILL ROGERS

Over the past few years I have been talk-ing—and writing—a lot about the changes in my life. Because I have shared

My good friend and former director of GMA *Bob McKinnon, guiding me through my first directing experience, Lindsay's music video. Dina Giordano, the choreographer, looks on.*

my experiences, other people want to talk to me about their lives, too. They want to be happier, healthier, thinner, richer, smarter, and many, many other *er's.* Their lives are filled with good intentions. I have emphasized that the first step in setting personal goals for

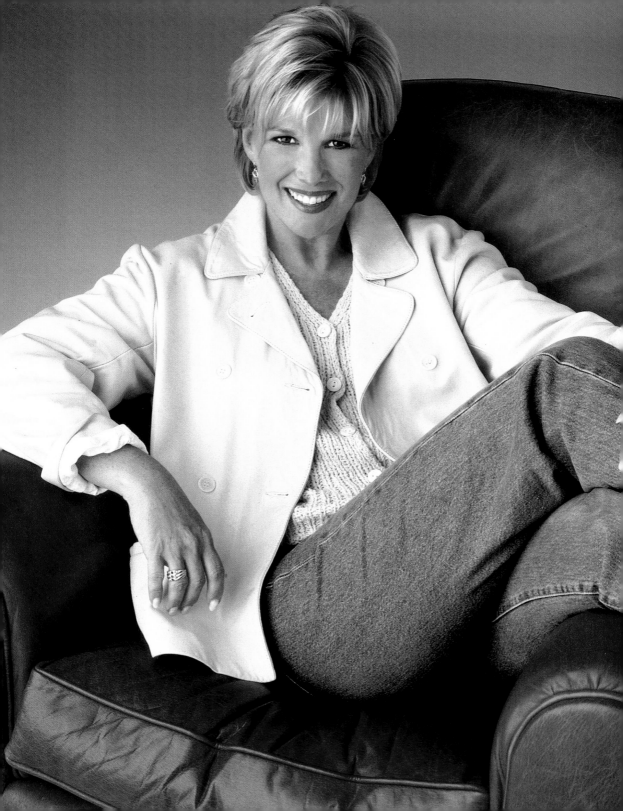

yourself is to reach one step further. You have to "just do it." The difference between those of us who change our lives and those of us who don't is first having the *desire* to change and then having the discipline to follow through. You have to put down all of those self-help books (except this one), stop watching infomercials late at night, and take action. Without action there can be no change.

> "My grandfather once told me that there are two kinds of people: those who do the work and those who take the credit. He told me to try to be in the first group; there was much less competition there."
>
> INDIRA GANDHI

Want to know the secret? Stop making excuses. Stop holding yourself back. Don't wait for your horoscope to tell you it's time.... Take charge, because it's *your* life and it's *your* decision. A lot of people have told me that they want to change but they're just too depressed or

they're just too busy. It's always too something. How many times have we all said, "I'll start that diet on Monday."? You have to stop waiting for those feelings to change all by themselves. You must change the way you think.

"Just do it" messages get sent to us every day. The point is to find something you enjoy and actively pursue it. Find something you're passionate about and take it one day at a time. When we were children, we enjoyed lots of activities. So why is it that as adults we think we have to give those things up? Well, we don't have to. Life is full of excitement and challenge, although it may come in many different forms and many different layers. Even when you think you know yourself, there is always another layer to peel away, revealing a new one underneath. This may sound a bit frightening—do we want to reach twenty or thirty or forty still wondering who we really are? But of course the flip side of fear is anticipation, and if we have the courage to admit it, we can be students of ourselves all our lives and love doing it. Some of our layers are really easy to uncover and identify, and some are more difficult. Over the years, I have discovered that each layer I unfold reveals just a little bit more of who I want to be and, even more important, who I really am.

Embrace Today

"Since you have to do the things you have to do, be wise enough to do some of the things you want to do."

MALCOLM FORBES

The idea of actually making an appointment with myself *for* myself was foreign to me. I was so busy seeing to the needs of my bosses, co-workers, friends, and family that I never had even a moment just for me. (Sound familiar?) Now, I love to make lists. I make lists of things I need to do, things I want to do, and even things to be crossed off my other lists! There was a time in my life when I would no sooner sit down and do nothing for an hour than have my fingernails pulled off one by one. Today I

have overcome my compulsive busyness, although I still need a reminder every now and then.

Take time to be friendly—
  It is the road to happiness.
Take time to dream—
  It is hitching your wagon to a star
Take time to love and to be loved—
  It is the privilege of the gods.
Take time to look around—
  It is too short a day to be selfish.
Take time to laugh—
  It is the music of the soul.

ANONYMOUS

Actively Participate in Your Life

As parents we spend a lot of effort urging our children to find a passion and be active in life. Part of that effort is to keep them fit, but it's also a way to help build their self-esteem. To help them find the youthful passion that we as

One of my favorite pictures: coming home from a horse show with Jamie.

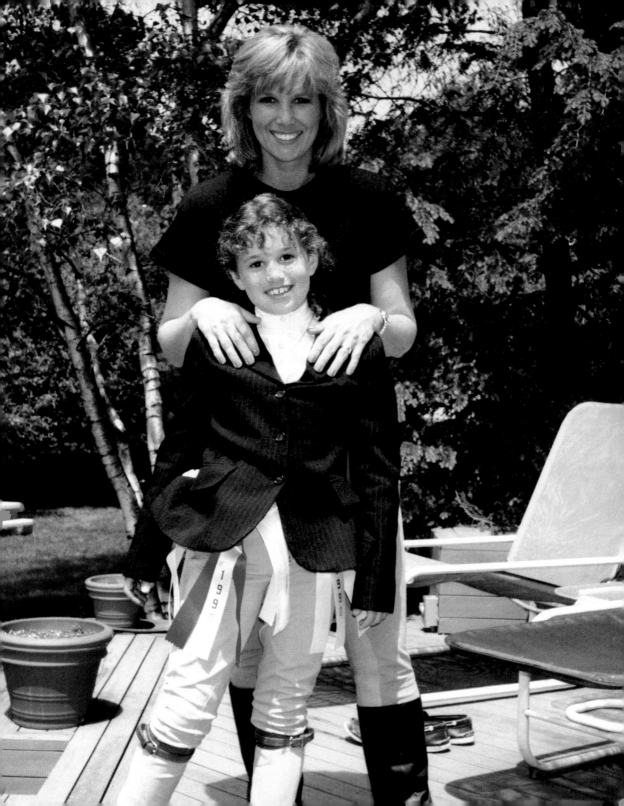

parents often look back on. I remember how, as a child, I was completely enthusiastic about horseback riding. So when my daughter Jamie was seven, I introduced her to the world of riding. (If only I had known then how much riding costs and the miles it would lead me to travel, I might have rethought that decision!) But Jamie took to this like a horse to hay. She fell in love with the sport, she absolutely adored her horses, and she embraced the competitive spirit. As they say, the apple doesn't fall far from the tree.

For almost a year I stood outside the riding ring, watching her as she delighted in the sport that had so inspired me as a child. I remembered riding at her age, galloping freely through the open fields near my home in Sacramento, with the wind blowing through my hair.

While I derived tremendous pleasure from watching Jamie excel and take pride in her sport, it took me a long time to acknowledge my own longing. Then one day it just hit me: I really missed riding, and I could think of no logical reason not to join Jamie in the ring. Maybe, I thought, it's like riding a bike....

But it wasn't, I'm sorry to say. And I didn't remember being that sore after riding as a kid. But after months of lessons and gaining confidence, my own competitive spirit once again reared its head. Not since the Judds has there been a better mother-daughter team. With our saddles loaded in the trunk of my car, we blazed a trail all over the Northeast, going from competition to competition.

I'm grateful that I allowed myself to recapture that part of my childhood, but I'm amazed that I had been so willing to deny myself that sense of play, that desire to embrace something so passionately. Why do we feel we have to do that?

The answer is that we don't have to. Walt Disney discovered this concept over forty years ago, when he opened Disneyland in Anaheim, California. His idea has grown into a multibillion-dollar business that has spread all over the world and endured for years. What it all boils down to is that Disney's fantasyland is your ticket to be a child again without guilt or embarrassment. You can allow yourself to enjoy the fantasy, the thrill, the excitement, and even to be scared. Disney recognized our desire to escape the complexities of our daily lives and recap-

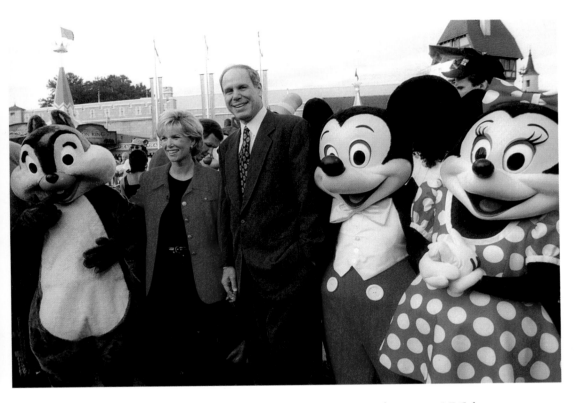

Here I am with my new ABC bosses, Michael Eisner, Mickey Mouse, and the board of directors.

ture the carefree days of our youth.

You can create magic in your own life, and, no, you don't need your own theme park. You need to give yourself permission to recall and revive your own childhood joys.

Start by asking yourself a few questions—and make a list of those answers! What was your passion as a child? Why aren't you pursuing it today? I asked myself, Why did I ever stop riding, anyway? Oh, yeah, I had to

go to college, date, get a job, date, move to New York, and date some more. You get the idea.

Dr. Ellen McGrath, a regular contributor on *GMA* and author of *When Feeling Bad Is Good,* explained to me the importance of rediscovering your passion as an adult: "The secret to aging successfully

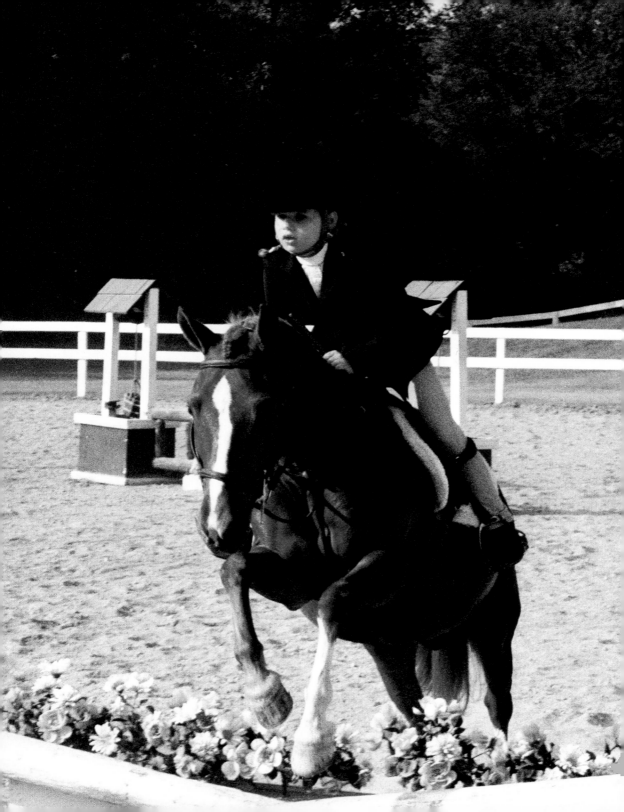

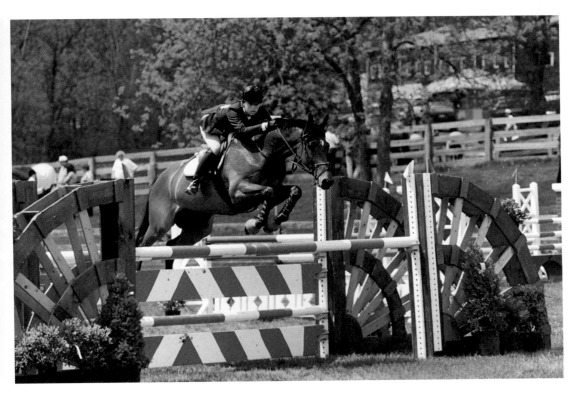

is to find and follow your passion. Passions are the interests that are so compelling and satisfying that we lose all sense of time as we pursue them. It could be getting lost in your rose garden, climbing Mount Kilimanjaro, or rediscovering a childhood passion like horseback riding or hiking."

Dr. McGrath is totally on the money. It's exactly the way I've felt since I got back in the saddle. As a bonus, riding has given me a special bond and sense of com-

OPPOSITE: *Jamie jumping at age seven.*
ABOVE: *Jamie jumping today at age sixteen.*

panionship with Jamie. Interestingly, exposing her to riding at an early age definitely accomplished my initial aims. Jamie learned discipline, the responsibility of caring for an animal, and how to win and lose gracefully. She also developed a healthy attitude toward competition and gained an enormous sense of self-esteem.

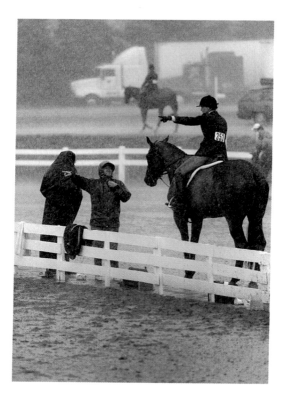

ABOVE: *Trainer Kip Rosenthal giving me last-minute instructions.* OPPOSITE: *When it rains, it pours.*

But it has become so much more. Taking up riding again provided me with a way to let go of everyday hassles, unwind, and have some good old-fashioned fun. Of course, some of my friends think that I have a pretty warped sense of fun when they see the lengths I'll go to ride. My most memo-

rable exploit to date occurred in a torrential downpour during the Lake Placid Horse Show, in upstate New York. This is a huge show with over a thousand horses competing. I attend with Jamie every summer. For a week I watched her compete in beautiful sunny weather, waiting for my chance, which didn't come until the last day, just about the same time that a huge black storm cloud rolled in right over the ring. I had already mounted and was waiting at the in gate when it started to pour. Within minutes, most of the other wimps pulled out of the competition, but I had waited all week for this opportunity, and I wasn't about to wimp out. My trainer, Kip Rosenthal, always a competitor, reminded me that as each rider dropped out, my chances of winning greatly increased. Of course she was laughing so hard she had a difficult time giving me my last-minute instructions. Undaunted, I entered the ring, and couldn't help laughing myself when the rain turned to hail somewhere between jump one and jump two. You may think it sounds crazy, but I won that ribbon and had a helluva lot of fun doing it, too! "Fun" is important in life,

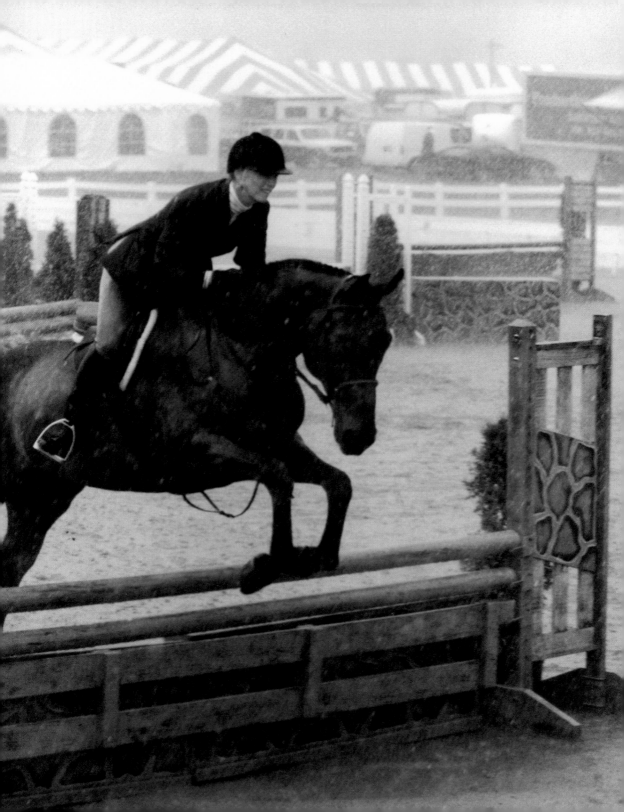

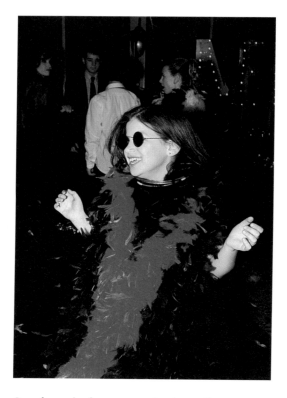

Sarah steals the scene on the dance floor.

and for a long time, maybe too long, I had forgotten that. I'm glad I rediscovered my passion.

Perhaps one of the best ways to learn to rediscover that sense of childhood playfulness is to watch your own children. My youngest, Sarah, has been one of my best teachers! She completely embraces the concept of no limits, and, boy, does she know how to enjoy each

moment of the day. Her sense of humor keeps us all in stitches. Maybe it's because she is the youngest of my three girls that she never lets fear hold her back from trying new things. She loves to emulate her big sisters. Like Lindsay, Sarah loves to dance—in fact, Lindsay is now the assistant teacher of one of Sarah's dance classes—and every summer Sarah goes off to camp at Pony Farm in New Hampshire to sharpen her riding skills, just like Jamie. And if there were more hours in the day, she'd probably host her own talk show, too!

Ironically, while we're busy trying to regain our youthfulness, our children can't wait to grow up. Sometimes Sarah's desire to be like her older sisters gets to be just a little too much. One day, when I asked the girls about their weekend plans, Sarah asked if I would drop her and her friend Charlie at the mall so they could have a bite to eat and go to the movies. To say that I was a little taken aback by this is the understatement of the year: my then eight-year-old seemed to be asking me if she could go out on a date! When I told her no, she said, "But, Mommy, Lindsay and Jamie do it all the time. Why can't I?" "Because you're eight years old, sweetie pie, and they're teenagers," I replied. Sarah seemed as surprised by my answer as I was by her question. I tried to explain my logic to her, but Sarah just kept saying that it wasn't fair!

I suppose that being the baby can be a blessing and a curse. They want the same privileges their older siblings have, but they still want to enjoy the benefits of being the baby. I think, for Sarah, it's still cool to hang out all day with me or her dad. Like most teenagers, Lindsay and Jamie have really established their own lives. The big challenge is keeping up with their social calendar. And for now I just love having Sarah still need me as a mommy and not just as a source for concert tickets, a chauffeur, or another closet to borrow clothes from. I'll tell you one thing I know for sure: in the middle of a hectic day, just the sound of her sweet little raspy voice over the phone is enough to put a smile on my face.

Strive to Be Happy

"Act as if you are already happy, and that will tend to make you happy."
DALE CARNEGIE

Finding reasons to be happy in your life is easier than you might think. It's the process of enjoying each moment to its fullest potential. What puts a smile on your face every time you think about it? Who do you enjoy being with? What setting makes you feel good? What makes you laugh? Make a point of looking for these moments in your life. Don't just wait around for them to fall into your lap. Even if you are struck in a traffic jam on the way to work, you can still plan a good meal, enjoy a great tune on the radio or CD player, or just appreciate the clouds in the sky. Create your own happiness.

Happiness means something different to everyone. To help get you started, here are some ideas. I know I smiled just thinking up the list.

- *Be an optimist.*
- *Have positive expectations.*
- *Have a voice.*
- *Learn to listen.*
- *Be honest and direct.*
- *Live in the moment.*
- *Don't wait for the future to bring you happiness.*
- *Laugh as often as possible —it makes you live better and longer.*
- *Enjoy the moments.*
- *Walk on the beach.*
- *Watch a sunset.*
- *Find your passions and pursue them.*
- *Honor your body and maintain your health.*
- *Speak openly about your feelings when you're angry or worried.*
- *Staying even is better than getting even.*

- *Be adventurous.*
- *Organize your time efficiently and effectively.*
- *List your priorities…and be true to them.*
- *Learn to say no—protect your time.*
- *Learn and be willing to delegate responsibility.*
- *Enlist support.*
- *Don't let procrastination bite ya in the butt!*
- *Set realistic goals and deadlines.*
- *Don't let fear of failure or criticism hold you back.*
- *Create a family of friends…a "safe place" to share feelings.*
- *Make quiet time for yourself each day to think and relax.*
- *Make exercise a permanent part of your life.*

- *Get enough sleep.*
- *Use deep breathing to relax and reduce stress.*
- *Make positive statements to yourself.*
- *Read and listen to inspirational and motivational material.*
- *Develop and nurture your creativity.*
- *Plant a garden.*
- *Smile and watch the world smile back.*
- *Look for the joy in your life.*
- *Be generous with your warmth and affection.*
- *Learn to recognize what you appreciate in your life, and it will give your life more meaning.*
- *Meditate—make an appointment with yourself.*
- *Listen to yourself.*
- *Believe in yourself.*
- *Connect with nature.*
- *Do something fun as often as you can get away with it.*
- *Enjoy the company of your children . . . while they're still children.*
- *Give yourself a break.*
- *Don't beat yourself up. Remember, you're only human.*
- *Indulge your inner child.*
- *Learn to love yourself—a necessity before you can love others.*
- *Invite loving relationships.*
- *Wish upon a star.*
- *Stop taking everything so personally.*
- *Dig your toes in the sand.*
- *Remain playful.*
- *Kiss and make up.*
- *Pamper yourself with a candlelit bath.*
- *Go dancing.*
- *Sing out loud in the car.*
- *Exude enthusiasm.*

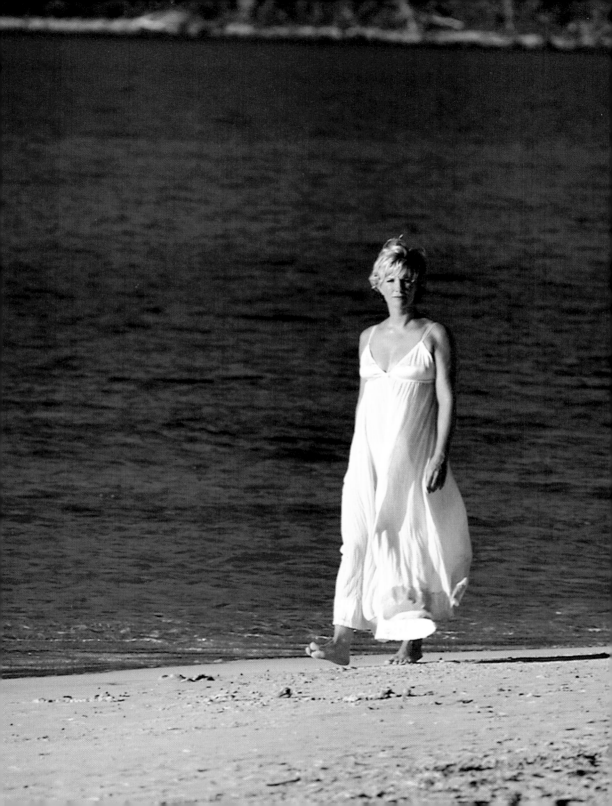

3 Becoming a Witness to Your Own Life

Becoming a witness to your own life means, quite simply, being able to take an honest look inside yourself. It means understanding how your inner being—the way your emotions affect everything you think and do—determines how you react to everyone and everything around you, even how you react to your own thoughts. Although you may not realize it, we have all had lots of practice at this activity—analyzing everyone *else*'s life. C'mon, admit it. I'll bet you've had a conversation with a friend or family member in the last week, trying to figure out just why Uncle Harry always jumps to conclusions and seems to be so defensive. Or how about that friend of yours who can't seem to make a relationship work? You might even have gone so far as to try to help others understand that their negative emotions were keeping them in a funk.

Then why is it so hard to accept that we have our own inner tensions? We too may be holding on to anger, resentment, or unresolved sadness, all of which can affect our thoughts and our reactions to everything around us. We all know we can't control what happens around us (though I've met a few people who thought they could!), but *we can control how we respond.* In the 1970s it was popular to speak of expressing your anger. A lot of people acted on this by telling off anybody they saw during the day—from the bank clerk to their spouses. Not only did all this sounding off upset some innocent bystanders, but it didn't make the people who were constantly expressing their anger feel that great, either. This is simply letting off steam; it is not dealing with the actual emotions.

Taking a look at your inner workings requires you to make some very honest assessments. If you're having a lousy day and every person you come into contact with can't wait to get out of your way, it's not them, it's you. If you find that you're constantly snapping at your husband, fighting over insignificant issues, and losing your patience, it's time to stop and ask yourself what is going on inside you. Do you have a lot of stored-up anger and resentment that is now coloring your interactions on a day-to-day basis? Wouldn't it be better to face your emotions and then be able to let go of them so that your relationships can become more enjoyable again?

And what about that teenager who won't give you the time of day anymore? Even though we know it's appropriate for kids that age to begin to break away from their parents, we still expect them to interact with us the way they did when they were youngsters. Expecting and wanting people to be the way *we* want them to be, instead of accepting them for who they are, is one of the negative "inner workings" that we all fall prey to. But not recognizing this can create adversarial, noncommunicative relationships and leave you feeling frustrated and upset. For example, if you take a deep breath or two or three and acknowledge that those teenagers are turning into their own individual selves, you may find your hurt and resentment turning into sympathy and wonder. And if that doesn't do it, you can always take away the car keys!

"We perceive, which means we add meaning to every signal coming our way."

DEEPAK CHOPRA

We've all heard the old saying "seeing the world through rose-colored glasses." The emotions that you carry around with you color the way you see things in life. Becoming a witness to your life means aspiring to see the world with a clear vision. It's not always easy. If we could leave our bodies for a week to watch ourselves from the outside objectively, it would make the process of self-realization a lot easier. I still haven't figured out how to master out-of-body travel (although I do have a call in to Shirley MacLaine!).

Inward investigation is like being your own psychoanalyst, figuring out what's making you feel bad, whether you're dissatisfied, angry, suspicious, or short-tempered. This kind of honest introspection can allow you to live with greater awareness, acceptance of others, and an overall harmony in your life. To avoid it means cheating yourself of potential happiness and opportunities for growth. Think of this process as an MRI, an X-ray of sorts, of your subconscious showing the calcifications that are the cause of your discomfort. Leaving these issues unattended over time will cause them to worsen until they seriously affect your overall health and mental well-being.

In a courtroom, a witness is an objective observer, and not a judge. Remember that your ultimate goal is to acknowledge, deal with, and let go of behavioral patterns that are holding you back from balanced growth and contentment. The idea here is not to beat yourself up. As a witness, you are merely there to observe and promote change, not defend your life.

Hollywood already made that movie. It starred Albert Brooks and Meryl Streep, and it really was called *Defending Your Life*. It told the story of two people (Albert and Meryl) who die and then must defend the way they lived in order to move on through the cycle of the universe or get sent back to earth to keep trying to reduce their karmic debt. The judging process is performed by making the characters watch film clips of their lives and then defend their actions to a council of judges. Albert's character has a lot more explaining to do than Meryl's. He must admit that he was a short-tempered, egotistical, defensive coward and then attempt to explain why he couldn't deal with his emotions and fears. Meryl Streep's character, on the other hand, was courageous, giving, and accepting of others. While the film is a comedy, it does pose some interesting questions. If you had to defend your life on earth, what areas would need the most explanation? Would you be the Albert Brooks character, who feared facing the truth about himself, or the Meryl Streep character, who took the higher road most of her life?

Take the Higher Road

We've all heard the saying "take the higher road" a million times before, but have you ever really stopped and thought about what it means and how to apply it to your life? It's one of the best lessons I have learned, and it came as an early Christmas gift in 1995.

Just before Christmas, I met my good friends Scot Evans and Laura Morton for coffee in lower Manhattan. We try to make it a point to get together before the craziness of the holiday season goes into full swing and we go off in our different directions to celebrate the New Year. Scot was headed to Palm Springs, California, for a meditation seminar celebrating life, happiness, and spirituality. Scot has worked hard to reach a high level of spiritual awareness and has taught me much of what I know about meditation. The conversation turned to our hopes and desires for the new year, both for ourselves and for each other. Laura and I made Scot go first, because quite frankly we knew he'd say something much smarter and deeper than either of us would, and we wanted to gauge our answers based on his. He said that all he wanted to do in the coming year was to "always try to take the higher road." Was I glad he went first! My thoughts were going down a totally different path, and I was about to wish for something far more superficial, like a handsome, sweet, loving, caring man in my life. But I decided that Scot's wish sounded like something much easier to achieve—sad but true.

I couldn't get over the impact his statement had on me. As the new year began, every time a tough situation cropped up, those four simple words, "take the higher road," entered my mind, and each time I followed that formula. It never once failed me. For me, taking the higher road means that sometimes—maybe even most of the time—you have to be the bigger person and make the first move. It eliminates the temptation to draw a line in the sand and make foolish mistakes out of pure stubbornness. We've all been there. You try to make a point, hold your position under fire, and finally turn something that might not have been such a big deal to start with into World War III! What makes us jump to conclusions or say things we will be sorry for later?

Sometimes it's really hard to step back and look at things clearly when your vision is clouded by emotions, but it is a necessary step to making smart decisions. Keep asking yourself questions about the motives behind your reactions and behavior. This kind of self-examination is the only thing that will lead to real change.

Looking Inside Yourself

Women's struggle to break free of the expectations and limitations put upon us by ourselves, our families, our employers, and society in general constantly makes us face ourselves in the mirror and evaluate how we're measuring up. But like Alice in Wonderland, you need somehow to get through that looking glass. I believe that most women have an insatiable thirst for knowledge and new ways to improve themselves. The process of educating oneself is the journey, but somewhat ironically the destination always remains unknown.

Several years back, I picked up magazines and read articles about women who were fabulous at forty, and I wanted so

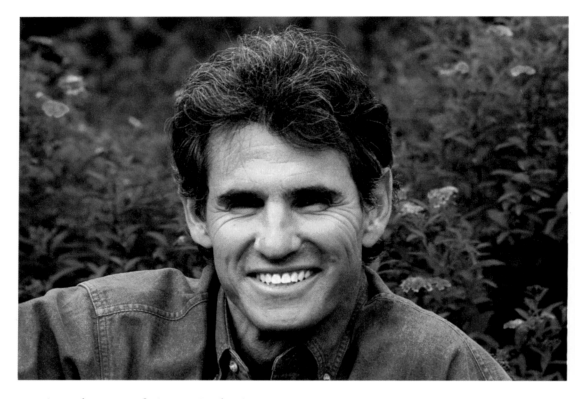

Jon Kabat-Zinn taught me to take a candid look inside myself.

much to be one of them. Back then I defined being fabulous at forty to mean looking great for your age and somehow finding a balance between the different areas of your life. Now I would add inner peace and serenity to that formula. Today I pick up magazines and the same fabulous-at-forty women are now becoming fantastic at fifty—Barbra Streisand, Goldie Hawn, and Bette Midler, to mention a few. But the best part for me is that today I am much closer to being

the kind of woman I admire. This took learning how to slow down, which was one of the toughest lessons for me, and learning to take an honest look at the things that made me happy and at those that made me sad. But in order to find the answers I had to learn to ask myself questions. The next chapter will help you learn how to ask yourself the right questions, so that you can understand your emotions.

Letting Go

I have a baseball hat collection that could probably be in the running for the *Guinness Book of World Records*. I have caps that say "Don't Go There," "Bad Hair Day," "Duh," "Get Over It," "Is It Friday Yet?" "What Goes Around Comes Around," "Talk Slow, I'm Blonde," and "Back Off." The list goes on and on, but I'm still looking for a hat that says "Let It Go." It's probably the most important message of all. I have come to the realization that if you can let go of things like anger and frustration, instead of losing control, you actually gain it. We're all afraid of releasing negative thoughts—as if they were some kind of precious jewels we have to hang on to, but letting go is the key to liberation. If you understand the basic principle of what "letting go" means, it will become a very powerful tool for growth and happiness.

The first time that I ever heard about letting go was when I read Jon Kabat-Zinn's *Wherever You Go, There You Are.* He gave two excellent analogies that really clarified this important concept:

Imagine letting your palm open to unhand something you have been holding on to tightly. Like your hand, we also hold on with our minds. By holding on, often desperately, to narrow views, fears, insecurities, and self-serving hopes and wishes, we stunt our ability to change and accept a new way of thinking.

Earlier in this chapter, I talked about how the emotions we carry around color the way we see things in life. Kabat-Zinn writes that all too often "we must allow ourselves to recognize the lenses we slip so unconsciously between observer and observed, that then filter and color, bend and shape, our view."

Another well-known inspirational novelist and writer, Toni Morrison, defines letting go about as bluntly as I've ever heard: "Wanna fly, you got to give up the shit that weighs you down."

Holding a *grudge* and harboring *resentment* are two of the most common emotions people have trouble releasing. This definitely gets in the way of building relationships with others. Remember that no matter what someone does to us, when we hold on to it, it hurts us, not them. Another old saying, "Forgive and forget," applies here.

Anger is an especially tough issue for women, because most of us are taught to hold anger in, while men are taught that it's acceptable behavior to let anger out. Additionally, women have so much on our plates, we're worn out most of the time. We tend to get angry when we're stressed out and exhausted. With this short fuse, we find ourselves snapping or yelling at those we love the most. Then, of course, we feel guilty and get angry at ourselves for being angry. Talk about a vicious cycle! While it's important to learn to deal with your anger, it's just as important to remember that anger is a human feeling, and all feelings, positive or negative, are normal. The issue really becomes a problem when we hold anger in, allowing it to build, and we find ourselves exploding on innocent people in a totally unrelated circumstance. Psychologists call this displaced anger, but your friends may just call you a bitch.

When it comes to *expectations,* I sometimes think of the words of a business adviser: "Expect *nothing* from anyone, and you'll never be disappointed."

Okay, so he's a little pessimistic and jaded, but the truth is, when we place expectations on others, we do run the risk of disappointment. People will not always respond to things the way we expect them to. And it's not just people who can let you down; it can even be something such as a social event. Haven't you ever gone to a party expecting it to be a particular kind of evening, and just because it didn't live up to your expectations all of the pleasure went out of the event for you? Conversely, we get ourselves into trouble trying to meet and live up to the expectations others place upon us. First of all, what are these expectations based on? Are they realistic? There's probably no group of people on earth who try harder than women to meet other people's expectations, since most of us were taught that our role in life is to nurture others. We're constantly looking outside ourselves for validation, but in trying to be what others think we should be, we lose who we really are in the process.

Ready for a biggie? Let's talk about *fear.* Fear can be paralyzing and can really hold you back. The definitions of fear run the gamut: fear that we're not good enough or smart enough, that we won't get our way, that bad things will happen, that good things won't last, that we're the only one in a group who doesn't know anything....

Jon Kabat-Zinn says that "this type of thinking dominates the mind and weighs it down. It's like carrying around a suitcase full of rocks on your head. It feels good to put it down."

Judgmental behavior comes in two forms. When you constantly judge others, they will tend to resent you or judge you in return. You may also fall victim to constantly judging yourself by evaluating yourself with an overly critical eye. Saying things like "I'm too fat" or "I'm too dumb" over and over will eventually make it true in your mind.

Control isn't exactly an emotion, but it is a need—our need to make other people think and behave as we want. And control freaks also tend to believe that it is their God-given right to do so, since they know everything, of course. Isn't it a little arrogant and even dis-

respectful to try to control the lives of others and tell them what's best for them? The need to control also weighs you down personally. It takes an enormous amount of time and energy, and it's a no-win goal. So get your need to control under control.

Letting go, despite the cliché, is not the process of allowing a harmful or unpleasant feeling, emotion, or thought simply to leave your mind. It is your ability to believe that you can change your negative perceptions. Simply put, you are letting go of the power these negative thoughts have over your life.

Shattering Self-Limits

"Courage is very important. Like a muscle, it is strengthened by use."
RUTH GORDON

Once you've started on your road to a happier, healthier life, you will find that it's time to challenge your self-limits. The concept of physical change is easy to understand and accept, because it's visible. Changes in your appearance can be gratifying because you, as well as others, can actually see those changes. I know this all too well—if I'm down ten pounds in my weight, believe me, it's noticed! If I change my hair, it's noticed. Sometimes these changes work, and sometimes when I look back, I wonder, What was I thinking?

An inner change is something you can't see as readily, and, maybe even more frustrating, it can be very gradual. (For those of you who are into instant gratification, sorry!) But it's just as important as physical change, if not more so. Learning to understand the connection between your body and your mind, and recognizing that they have a powerful effect on each other, will help you discover your own path to a happier, healthier life without any self-imposed limitations.

Limits—just the word itself is limiting. There are limits that are mandated for our own good, such as speed limits, and then there are limits that we unfairly place upon ourselves. Why is it that we, as women, have a tendency to be so hard on ourselves? We're usually our own toughest critics, and most of

the time to a fault. Most of us will automatically set limits for everything that we do. If you were to do sit-ups, how many do you think you would do? Ten? Twenty? Thirty? No matter what your answer is, I assure you that it is a nice even number. But what happens when you get there? Do you quit just because you've hit the goal? We make up our minds that we can only do a certain number, and that is where we stop. The same theory can be applied to many areas of your life. While setting goals is a positive step for reinforcement, be careful not to limit your potential by setting them too low or stopping at the goals without considering whether or not you could surpass them. Next time you do sit-ups, go for as many as you can, and then do one more.

The idea that you can push yourself just a little bit further next time is unthinkable to many people, but it is essential to growth. That's not to say that there aren't boundaries, whether they're physical, emotional, or professional, and I'm not suggesting that you cross boundaries that would take you into dangerous territory, whether it's a mountain too high to climb or an area so

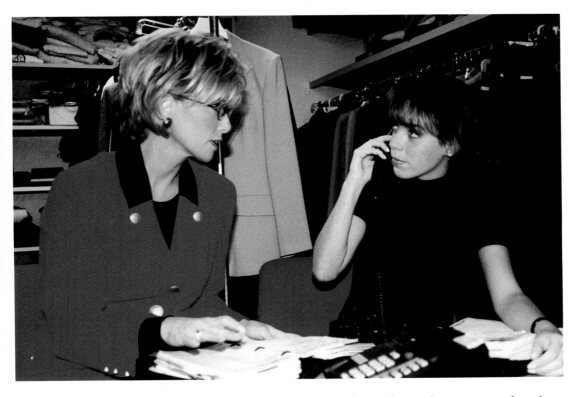

Jill is always there to keep me on track and on time.

far outside your expertise that you would jeopardize yourself or others. Believe me, when I was climbing the Tetons, that concept was never clearer. And, in my everday professional life, I have to constantly tell myself not to be too ambitious in making commitments. Luckily my wonderful assistant, Jill Alpert Seigerman, is always near to remind me when I'm getting overzealous with my schedule.

But it's an important life lesson that

no matter what stage of life you are in, it doesn't take a mountain to shatter your own self-limits. I learned this lesson for the first time when I came to New York to work for WABC-TV. Back in Sacramento, at KCRA-TV, I had started out as the weather girl and consumer reporter, but I quickly moved right into an anchor position. While

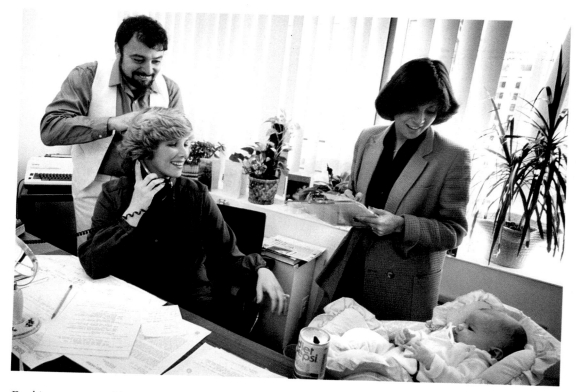

Booking guests and burping babies—all in a day's work in my first few months at GMA, *with twenty-two-year-old Elise Silvestri.*

anchoring is an ultimate goal in broadcast news, the stations' fervor to get women anchors on the air in those days meant that I missed gaining the experience of being a street reporter. So now here I was in New York City, first day on the job, and I was sent to the New York Supreme Court to cover a bombing and conspiracy trial. I didn't want anyone to know that I had only been inside a courtroom once...and that was to fight a traffic ticket. Thank goodness for my camera crew that day. They gave me a crash course in urban journalism, and I was able to make the story work, even though it took a few takes. That was definitely a day when I pushed the boundaries of my own self-limits.

Sometimes, if you're lucky, shattering your own self-limits will have an impact on someone else's life. That happened to me when I moved to the hosting position on *GMA*. It was one of the happiest times of my life, not just because of the great new job but also because I found out that I was pregnant with my oldest daughter, Jamie, the day I started. When I gave birth to her in 1980 I didn't want to miss out on the joys of being a new mother, so I became the first national television host to negotiate bringing my baby to work with me as part of my contract. In fact, ABC-Television executives provided me with an extra dressing room that became Jamie's baby room, complete with a changing table and crib. I would finish doing the show, and Elise Silvestri, my assistant at the time, and I would shuffle Jamie back to my office and work the rest of the day. Jamie had a swing in my office, and everyone would stop by for a little Jamie "fix." Today many companies are providing on-site day care for their employees. And by the way, that very same Elise Silvestri, who pushed the swing and burped Jamie and changed her diapers, is today a working mother who brings her kids to the office on occasion. And since she's part of the writing team

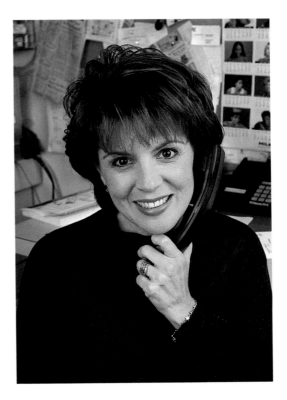

Elise is now a senior producer at the Sally Jessy Raphael *show.*

who put this book together, we've all taken turns burping and swinging her little ones. Fair is fair.

But juggling a career and a new baby was not the only challenge in my early days at *GMA*. If ever there was a time of true trailblazing for women in the media, that was it. Even though we woke up at four in the morning, worked

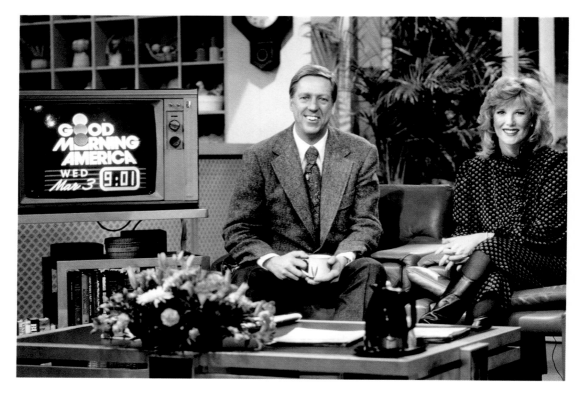

Early days on GMA *with David Hartman.*

the same hours, and diligently studied for our interviews, in those days the female morning television hosts took home significantly less money and served merely as props on the set. I remember a *Time* magazine cover featuring David Hartman, my co-host at the time, holding a little gift box containing a caricature of me. In fact, Jane Pauley (who was doing the *Today* show) and I

were both presented as perky little gifts for our male co-hosts. *Saturday Night Live* would do spoofs of our show, with Joe Piscopo doing his impression of David Hartman while I was depicted as a blow-up doll. It wasn't easy in those days. Constantly being barraged with this media perspective that my role was insignificant, I had to struggle not to fall into the trap of seeing myself that way, too. But to buy into someone else's view of me would have meant setting

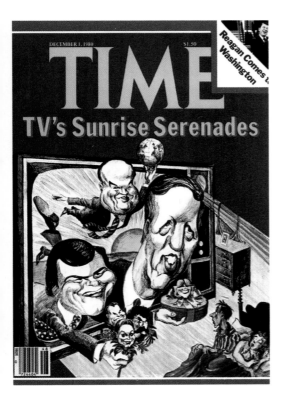

Boy, have times changed!

self-limits. It took patience, perseverance, and belief in myself to turn a deaf ear to stories that included statements such as "He gets Richard Burton, she gets an expert on head lice"—*TV Guide,* June 1983.

I have to laugh a little when I think about those days, though I understood my role at the time. I remember a piece of advice that Barbara Walters once gave me. She said, "Whatever they give you, make it a golden nugget." So I learned to pan for gold in my career.

Shattering self-limits can immeasurably boost your self-image. As you make progress, you can't help but feel better about yourself. Don't be afraid of failure; it will help you learn for next time. Try to picture yourself in the future, accomplishing whatever it is you set out to do. Twenty years later I'm still on *GMA* and loving it. These days I'm the veteran of morning television, and the roles of male and female host are equal. By applying the same techniques of perseverance and positive thinking, I still find that the show constantly provides me with ways to grow and challenge myself.

When *GMA* went to Aspen in February of 1996, I realized they were expecting me to ski down the mountain with my co-host, Charlie Gibson, to open the show. I hadn't been on skis since I covered the 1976 Olympics in Sarajevo! What if I fell? I couldn't afford the time to be injured.

But I was to find this skiing adventure a unique experience. There, at the top of Aspen Mountain, where I

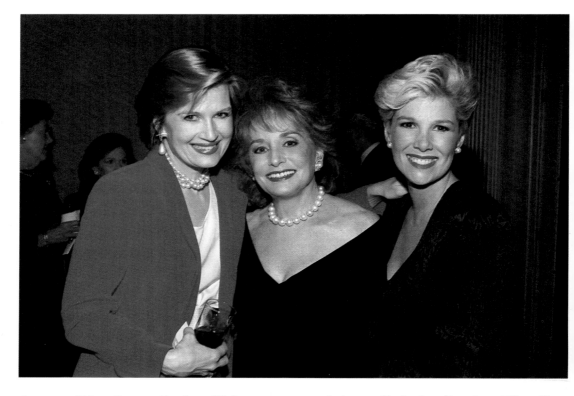

ABOVE: *Diane Sawyer, Barbara Walters, and me at an ABC awards dinner.* OPPOSITE: *Two of my best buddies—Charlie Gibson and Spencer Christian.*

expected I'd be nervous and tentative, I discovered something quite different.

Drawing on my newfound sense of confidence, fit body, and positive attitude, I decided to try a new approach to this sport. I have interviewed countless athletes who use a technique in their training called visualization. Visualization is simply mentally seeing yourself performing the task or sport at hand like a pro. Years ago I had always skied cautiously, traversing each hill endlessly back and forth and back and forth, constantly saying to myself, "Oh, please, God, don't let me fall. Don't let me fall." On this day I decided to approach skiing differently. Before this moment, visualization had just been a theory, but as I stood there on

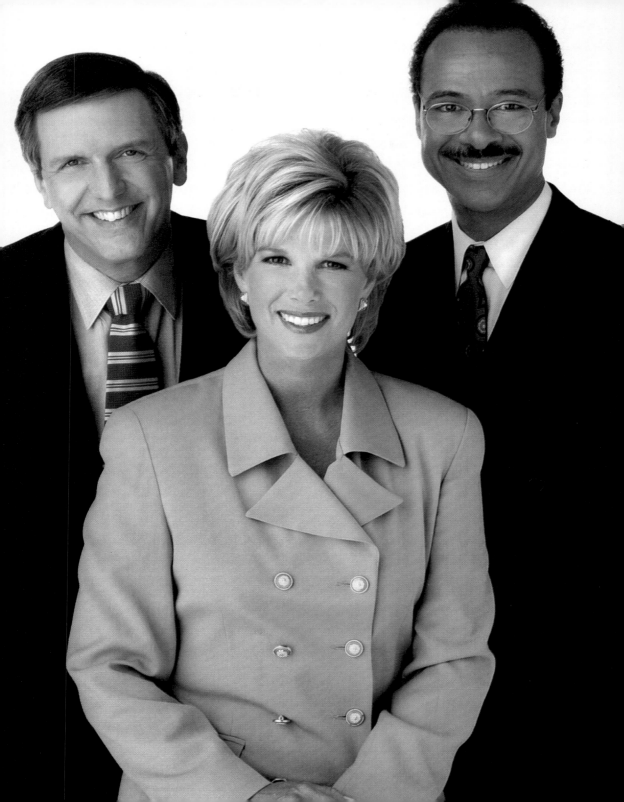

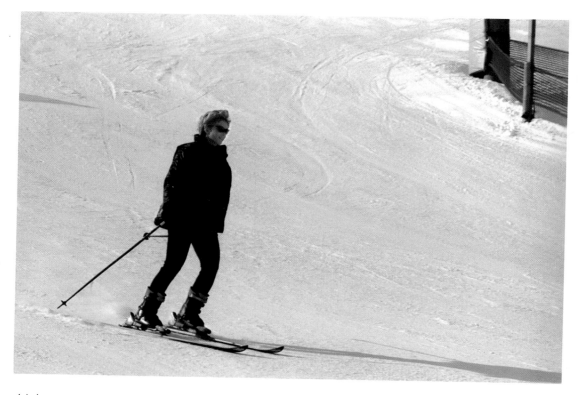

Ain't no mountain high enough...loving it in Aspen, Colorado.

Aspen Mountain, I imagined myself in perfect form, relaxed, never questioning my balance or the possibility that I might fall. I saw myself gliding down the mountain, cutting back and forth through the light powder snow, with barely any effort on my part. I pushed off down the trail, and it was the most amazing experience. My skis were perfectly parallel as my relaxed body acted like a shock absorber to the lumps and dips of the terrain. Employing the techniques of visualization and positive self-input, I found myself skiing just as I had envisioned—and as I had never skied before. I was shushing down Aspen Mountain like all of those people I used to watch from the chairlift and never thought I could be. It was an extremely freeing and fun experience, and I had almost missed it entirely. That

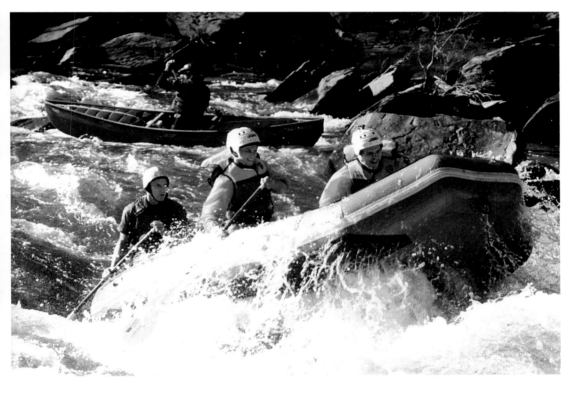

Ain't no river wide enough...Charlie and me white water rafting on another exciting GMA adventure.

silly game of "what if" almost held me back. "What if I fall?" or "What if I can't do it?" You've probably played the "what if?" or "what's the worst thing that could happen?" game a million times, too. But it's really a senseless game that wastes your time, drains your energy, and greatly limits your potential.

The opposite of the "what if" game is the "I believe I can do anything" game. It's easier if you play with a team that has the same belief in you. When de-

ciding what to do with my *Behind Closed Doors* specials on ABC, it was no accident that I chose a vehicle that allowed me to try new things, like flying F-18 jets, training with the Navy SEALs on nuclear submarines, tagging along on FBI and CIA missions, and appearing onstage with musical sensa-

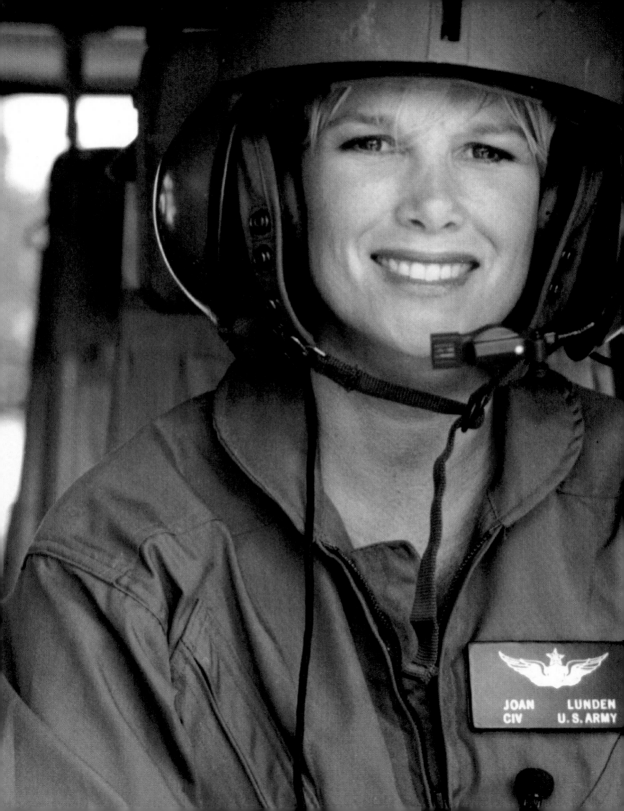

tions Michael Bolton and Celine Dion. These specials have become a ticket to adventure for me. I constantly hear from people, "I can't believe you did that!" Okay, I'll admit it, sometimes when we first discuss venturing into uncharted territory to try to get behind yet another closed door, I too wonder, "Can I really do that?" Part of my secret has been surrounding myself with a team that truly believes there's nothing I can't do. I have actually thought to myself, "I wish I believed in me as much as my incredibly talented and unbelievably optimistic producers, Eric Schotz and Bill Paolantonio, do." I've learned that I can feed off of their positive energy to make myself better at my game.

People usually think of shattering self-limits in terms of taking a few strokes off their golf game, finally beating that opponent in tennis, or getting a promotion at work. But rarely do we recognize that we can also shatter emotional self-limits. This can mean learning how to communicate better with a

Flying in restricted air space above the nation's capital, preparing to land at the Pentagon.

spouse or perhaps learning to overcome the fear of confrontation. I found it can even mean discovering a new depth within yourself.

When I visited the Golden Door Spa in December 1995, I experienced a lot of personal breakthroughs. Believe it or not, it was the first time that I had gone on vacation by myself, not to mention my first experience with hiking. And it was my first real accomplishment in expressing my feelings and emotions. I have always marveled at my daughter Jamie's ability to tell people—straightforwardly and simply—exactly how she feels. Since age four she's been able to capture her feelings beautifully in writing, especially poetry. I always wondered where she got that gift, but I have learned that we all have many gifts, but we must allow ourselves to unwrap them.

Before I left New York for the Golden Door, Scot, with his usual spiritual encouragement, suggested that I keep a pen and paper handy just in case I felt the urge to capture my feelings on paper. The mere suggestion actually unnerved me. And yet I must say that all of the experiences at the spa—push-

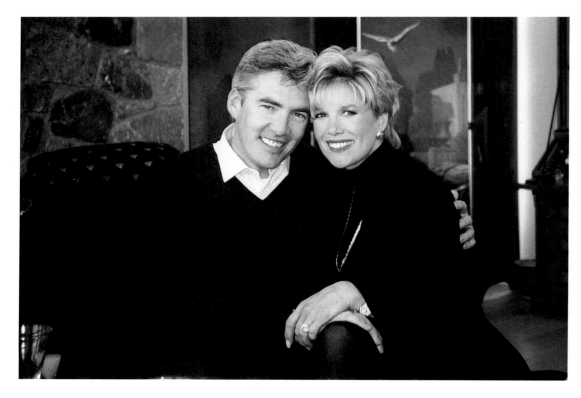

My soul mate, Scot Evans.

ing my limits of physical endurance, allowing my anxieties to float away during massage and meditation—really did promote the feeling of a safe haven for expressing my thoughts. In fact, once I embraced this idea, it was as if the floodgates had opened, maybe for the first time in many years.

Halfway through the week I woke up in the middle of the night and sat straight up in bed. A poem was just falling out of my head. Where was this coming from? In fact, who was this talking? I was afraid that if I didn't grab a pen and capture it quickly, I would forget it by morning, especially since it was for the very person who had suggested keeping the pen and paper handy. I scribbled the following words, which seemed to come from a place deep inside me, a place I never knew existed:

FOR A SOUL MATE

Oh, how precious to have a friend like
* you,*
Always there to share your excite-
* ments, your triumphs, and your*
* pain and anger too.*
Never too busy to lend your ear,
Always there to calm my fear.
Void of judgment, jealousy, resent-
* ment, or control,*
Only the purest of friendship that
* comes from deep in the soul.*
Walking through this life, knowing
* that you're there,*
And no matter how my day goes,
I find solace that you care.
I only hope and pray,
That I can be such a friend to you
* each day.*
But in you I derive the strength and
* courage to go deeper inside,*
And only there does this kind of gift
* reside.*
I know now that I will reach that
* enlightened land,*
Because I'm walking with you hand
* in hand.*

I know that it seems like a simple task to tell someone close to you how you feel about him, but it has never been easy for me. Just to be able to write down my feelings and have them remotely reflect how I was feeling was a tremendous achievement. It broke a self-limit that I had unfairly put on myself and one that I couldn't be happier to have broken. Recognizing the limits that you have imposed is the first step toward change. You must be willing to leave that comfort zone you have created for yourself and take risks.

Empowerment from Letting Go

If you let go of the power that negativity has over you, your highest unencumbered self will become the source of all your power. Your backbone will be strong, and negative energy will not weigh you down.

During times of crisis you must deal with, and let go of, many pent-up feelings. These are times when you find yourself questioning much in your life. You look inside and outside yourself to try to find the answers. You witness yourself going through incredible change, and you try to decide how best to deal with it. Like many people, I went through a time like this.

I made one of the most difficult decisions of my life when I decided to get a divorce. I had to take that very uncomfortable, scary, and sad step that would change my life forever. Filled with so much emotion, divorce takes on a life of its own. Issues that should be simple to resolve become emotionally charged. My need to defend my position was heightened by the fact that my divorce was scrutinized and exploited by the press. Though your friends and family are well intentioned, they too fuel the fire when they voice their support for "your side." Ultimately, they feed your feelings of anger and resentment.

Amid all this turmoil, I received an unexpected but much needed call from Michael Bolton, whom I had interviewed many times over the years. His friendly advice came from his own experience, and he shared it with me in the hope that it would ease my pain: "I've been down the road that you are about to walk down, Joan. It's not a pleasant journey, and you want to make it as

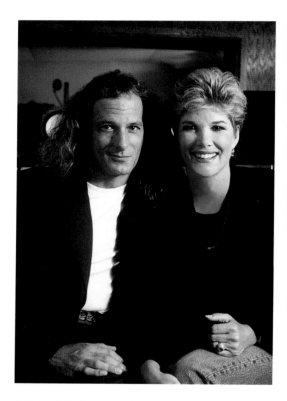

Michael Bolton—a friend I can lean on.

short as possible." He told me that the longer I allowed this to drag on, the more intense things would get, and I would become paralyzed by anger and hurt. He knew I was feeling as if I couldn't move on, but he urged me to push ahead as quickly as possible. Michael explained the dangers of letting other people talk me into "evening the score," which would obstruct me from letting go so I could get back on my feet again. I realized that he was telling me this not only for my sake but for my children's sake as well. Michael also has three daughters, and he knows the importance of bringing closure, peace, and harmony into your life again.

While his words obviously became emblazoned in my mind, so much so that I remember them verbatim today, it was really hard to act on them when I was in the thick of things. I knew Michael was right, though, and I finally decided that the only way to go was to take the higher road. I would not try to even the score. It was more important for everyone involved to start to heal.

The healing process took longer than I thought it would, but it would have taken even more time if I had not let go. Holding on to anger, resentment, and hurt only gives you tense muscles, a headache, and a sore jaw from clenching your teeth. It tires you out and wears you down. These emotional thieves rob you of time that you could spend being happy and having fun. When you finally get out from under that cloud and let go of all those negative feelings, it is the most empowering feeling you can ever know. Having the ability to let go and find forgiveness gives you back your laughter and the lightness in your life. A heart filled with anger has no room for love. . . .

I love life today.

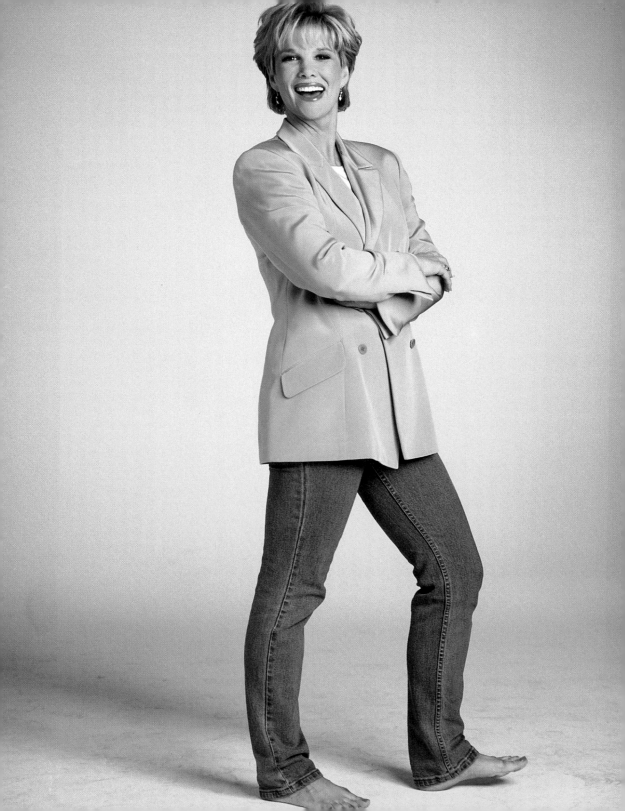

4 Power Thinking

A happy person is not a person in a certain set of circumstances, but rather a person with a certain set of attitudes.

—HUGH DOWNS

W e learn more and more every day about how our attitudes and our outlook have a tremendous effect on the way our bodies function. For me, the number one requirement for attaining a healthy mind and body is maintaining a positive attitude. Researchers in both the psychological and medical fields say that optimism is a major determining factor in our level of fitness. In fact, their research shows that optimism can help prevent disease and contribute to the healing process,

ADVICE FROM MY MOTHER

1. Have a party at least once a year to clean out your house.
2. Tan fat looks better than white fat.
3. Give others gifts you'd like to get yourself.
4. When you fight with your mate, don't tell your mother or your best friend, because you'll forgive and forget, but they'll always remember what a jerk he was.
5. Always reach for the stars.

whereas pessimism can seriously erode health. It's that old mind-over-matter thing.

Positive input and positive reinforcement were sprinkled throughout my childhood by my own personal guru— my mother, Gladyce. She constantly shared positive thoughts, such as "The word 'impossible' is not in my dictionary," and "There's no such word as 'can't.'" As a youngster, I always thought that my mom was the world's greatest and wisest philosopher. It's only in recent years that I discovered her pearls of wisdom date back as far as Napoleon, who said, "The word impossible is not in my dictionary."

Mom has always had an unbelievable ability to look on the bright side, a trait that couldn't always have been easy. Losing my father when my brother Jeff and I were twelve and thirteen, respectively, and having to go it alone as a parent during our teenage years must have been a challenge for her. She knew what a strong influence my father had always been, and now it was up to her and her alone to instill in us high goals and a positive atti-

With my mom.

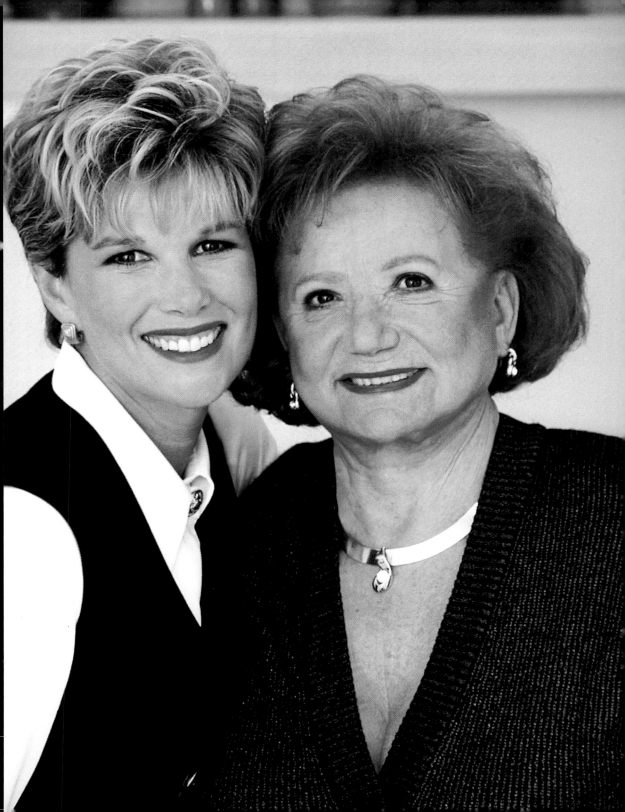

tude. Being the little independent soul that I am and always was, I argued, defied, and pushed every limit. (My mother always said, "Someday I hope you have a child just like you"…and now I do!) But Mom persevered and was relentless in her efforts to set a good example, build character, and give us confidence. Ultimately she taught me to believe in myself, and because of that when I set out to accomplish something, I succeeded.

Mom went to great lengths to provide opportunities that would open our eyes to all of the wonderful opportunities in the world to expand our horizons. And because she gave me faith in myself and a sense that I could accomplish anything I tried, I can now pass that feeling of empowerment on to my daughters.

If you can pass the gift of optimism on to others, they will benefit from it too. Unfortunately, living in today's world, it's almost too easy to be a pessimist. It's hard enough to face everyday obstacles, let alone believe that we can make a difference in these complex times. The world seems to be out of control, and that makes us feel powerless. Although life presents us with a lot of events that are beyond our control, we can still con-

trol how we respond to them. Our attitudes determine how we view and respond to life's events and challenges.

Positive Thinking, Positive Results

"We are the only creatures on earth who can change our biology by what we think and feel."

DEEPAK CHOPRA

How many times have you worked yourself into near panic simply by letting your thoughts run away with you and mentally creating a situation that does not exist? This tendency seems to be most prevalent in women, because we certainly know how to emotionally beat ourselves up. Why are we so quick to take the blame when our guy is in a terrible mood, the kids have the flu, or it snows only on our days to drive the carpool? When you are depressed, you feel lethargic, tired, grumpy, maybe even physically sick. But when you are happy, you automatically feel light, carefree, and energetic. So it makes sense that your attitude can set the tone for your well-being.

Optimists are known to be healthier than pessimists because they take an active role in their own personal health. They are more likely to have an exercise routine, eat properly, and regularly see a doctor. According to Martin Seligman, author of *Learned Optimism,* studies have shown that people who are frequently angry, suspicious, and mistrustful are twice as likely to develop coronary disease. Pessimism is a learned response; pessimists take every negative comment personally, jump to conclusions, and worry constantly—but they were hardly born with these traits. Just as you have to exercise your body to have good muscle tone, you have to exercise your positive attitude to keep it fit. And just as with physical exercise, the results of mental exercise are well worth the effort.

Not too long ago a friend of mine was talking to me about a situation involving her daughter. Her little girl had planned a play date with a friend and insisted on canceling out at the last minute. My friend was convinced that the other child's mother was going to be angry with her for allowing her daughter to cancel the plans, so she avoided seeing or talking to the woman for weeks. It turned out that the other mother wasn't mad at all, and my friend had wasted countless precious hours worrying about it and delaying a resolution of the situation. Here again anticipation robs you of the opportunity of experiencing the moment. How much easier it would have been if she had faced the other mother immediately, apologized, and discovered what the situation truly was before she reacted to it, saving herself a lot of aggravation and wasted energy.

We've all been there. You call someone or bump into an old friend at a restaurant, and the person seems kind of distant and abrupt. Inevitably, you hang up the phone or walk away, wondering to yourself, "What did I do?" Nine times out of ten you did nothing at all! Usually it turns out your friend was preoccupied with a problem of her own. Many studies show that women are more likely to blame personal qualities for failure, while men are far more likely to blame outside factors, like the weather. That cycle of self-blame and guilt freezes your ability to feel good about yourself. And if you're a real perfectionist like me, you can take self-blame to new heights. I have high standards and expectations for myself, so if I sometimes fall short of possibly overzealous goals, I tend to perceive it as a failure in some way. Thinking like this all the time is totally unfair and unnecessary. Analyzing an event or interaction is constructive if you learn from it and use it to bolster your self-awareness, but overanalyzing can become detrimental. You can learn to be an optimist if you make the effort to become aware of the negative thoughts and responses that jump into your mind uninvited. But you also can reprogram your way of thinking—with more realistic, constructive, and accepting attitudes.

Simple Ways to Build a Positive Attitude

- Constructive change happens when you take a positive direction in your life. This may sound simple—in fact, almost so easy that it's too good to be

true. I actually took a class on positive self-input, which is often referred to as positive self-talk or sometimes affirmations. You literally tell yourself how you want to feel. In this class we were taught to think uplifting thoughts at night as we were going to sleep, and again in the morning as we were starting our day. What we said was not so important as how, and there was really only one rule: Never use a negative word while practicing affirmation.

Don't say, "I won't get more than four hours of sleep tonight, but I'll make it feel like eight." Instead, say, "For the next four hours I'm going to have the deepest, most restful sleep. My body will generate fresh new cells, and I'll feel like a million bucks in the morning. I'll bound out of bed, feeling refreshed and renewed. I'll have such a sparkle in my eyes and such a bright smile on my face that I'll make everyone else smile."

Has this worked for me? All too often I have to make do with five or six hours of sleep—even less when I have a 3:45 wake-up call. But tell me, do you see a tired, grouchy face greet-

DAILY REMINDERS FOR A POSITIVE LIFE

◆ *Today I will search for my own identity and better define what I stand for.*

◆ *Today I will give some of the best of myself to others.*

◆ *My body is healthy, strong, and vibrant.*

◆ *Today I have the power to change what needs to be changed in my life.*

◆ *Today I will listen to myself as well as to others.*

◆ *Today I will trust in myself.*

◆ *I will look for the joy in this day.*

◆ *I'm a problem-solver, not a victim.*

◆ *Today I will stop reacting to everything.*

◆ *Today I will claim some time for myself.*

◆ *Today I will accept people for who they are and not who I want them to be.*

◆ *Today I will change what I can and accept what I can't change.*

◆ *Today when I'm overwhelmed by responsibilities, I'll think of one thing at a time and concentrate on changing or altering that one thing.*

◆ *Today I will broaden my own horizons.*

ing you at 7:00 each morning on *GMA*? You bet it's worked for me, and it can work for you, too.

◆ Focusing on the positive things in your life will help you cope with whatever challenges come your way. We're so used to focusing on our endless lists of things to do that sometimes it's easier to see what we haven't done than it is to see what we have done. So here's your exercise: Make a list of all the good things in your life—things you have accomplished, things you do well, and things to be thankful for. Stop and take stock every now and then. You may miss the opportunity to marvel at your wonders because you're so busy concentrating on, or grousing over, all that you still have left to do. Creating lists like this and making encouraging statements about yourself, to yourself, may sound kind of strange, and at first you will probably feel self-conscious about doing it. But this can actually make an imprint on your subconscious mind and create a healthy, positive self-image.

◆ Experts, from food and nutrition professional Jane Brody to Deepak Chopra, are also telling us that we must be able to see our life the way we want it before we can change, and the same goes for our bodies. This is another form of visualization. If you understand that your feelings and your behavior are greatly affected by your internal images, then you have a powerful tool for better health and greater happiness.

Not only that, but truly believing that things are great in your life will send that same message to those around you. It'll make all of those other people say, "I want what she's having." How you project yourself is how others perceive you as well. If you exude vitality and warmth, you will find that people will respond in a positive way. If your tone is short and demanding, watch out, because you're likely to elicit a similar attitude in return.

Creating a comfortable and happy self-image and applying it to your everyday routine will in turn affect each and every thing you do and everyone you touch. You can do anything when you take charge of your thoughts. And that's the ultimate irony: if you set out to control others you will surely fail, but if you get control of yourself, the behavior of others will change.

◆ Reading inspirational and educational messages and listening to them in person or on CDs will inspire positive thoughts. Think of it as one more way to exercise and condition your attitude. Every time I walk into a bookstore, I am invariably drawn to the inspirational books, and I find that they continually renew my spirit.

◆ Surround yourself with positive people. This may seem obvious, but it is so important that it bears repeating. Without realizing it, we absorb a great many emotional vibrations from the people we spend time with. The stronger the emotional bond to the other person, the greater effect those vibrations have on our lives and our emotions. If they build up over a long period of time, they can actually have a negative effect on our minds and bodies.

◆ Learn to ask yourself better questions. This is one of the most powerful tools that I have found for raising my self-awareness. But it was also one of the hardest exercises for me to learn and accept. Asking questions of yourself can help you in several different ways. In a time of crisis when much is required of you, you can choose how you will respond by choosing the questions you present to your brain. Instead of asking "Why does this always happen to me?" ask "What can I do to improve this situation?" or "What can I learn from this so that it won't happen again?" Learning to ask the right questions can be very enlightening.

Exercises like these may sound simple or silly until you actually try them. Have you asked yourself lately what about your life makes you happy? What you're grateful for? Whom you love? Who loves you? You'd be surprised at how listening to the answers can provide you with more happiness, more contentment, and more excitement in your life.

◆ Set positive goals for yourself. It's important to state your goals without using negative words like "don't," "won't," and "can't." Setting achievable goals and accomplishing them will help raise your self-esteem and generate a great attitude. This will help you feel better about yourself and also influence how others perceive you. When I set out to lose all of those extra pounds at age thirty-nine, I wanted immediate results. I had to learn to create a series of small achievable goals that I could meet and feel successful about, which boosted my self-confidence. That gave me the incentive to try for the next level. Take the time to acknowledge short-term successes, and the long-term goals will follow.

◆ Create healthy mind chatter. Mind chatter is that little voice inside your head that keeps you up at night fretting about your job, your bills, your kids. It's also the voice that analyzes, judges, and guides each and every move you make. This voice can empower you or hold you back. It can build confidence or tear it down. Learning to allow only positive mind chatter will help you empower yourself.

A great technique to help clear your head of negative mind chatter is described by Deepak Chopra in *The Way of the Wizard*. Deepak describes negative mind chatter as all of those worries of the day, plus a few bonus worries we think of that bog us down. He suggests allowing these stressful, irritating questions to come into your mind but to let them go just as quickly. Visualize those thoughts literally drifting upward out of your head, out of your bedroom, and far, far away. See them fly out of your mind just as quickly as they dropped in uninvited. What rude guests!

With all that I've said up to this point about positive thinking and always trying to look on the bright side, I concede that there will indeed be some days that will get the best of you. With my hectic schedule, there are days when I find myself overcommitted and my patience is tested. I may have put tremendous thought and preparation into the planning of that day, and then everything just seems to fall apart. Maybe my alarm doesn't go off, or it does but I fall back to sleep. I might be late for work, which means that I have less time to prepare for the show that morning. Inevitably, those are the mornings when we have a lot of technical difficulties on the show, or a guest cancels at the last minute, and every interview is like pulling teeth. As my day continues to unfold, I realize that I have double-booked myself for lunch, I'm going to be late picking up my girls at school, and the plumber hasn't returned my call about fixing the sink that has been clogged since dinner last night, and I haven't even thought about what's for dinner tonight. Well, I could go on and on, but I think you know where I'm going. After all, Momma said there'd be days like this!

These are the days—and thank goodness they're pretty few and far between—when I have to try to keep my perspective steady and my anxiety level at a dull roar. There's no avoiding it: these days will happen. I always think that someone up there must have a hell of a sense of humor to test me in this way: "Let's see how much I can pile onto Joan today." Hey, I've been weight training, but the weight of the world is still a little beyond my reach—you know what I mean?

Negative Thinking: The Emotional Thief

When you wake up, does just thinking about your day make your stomach knot up? "Which child has a play date after school? What's the deadline for summer camp sign-up? What am I making for dinner tonight? Did I remember to pick up the dry cleaning? There's no way I'm going to be able to do everything I need to do today!" If you start your day this way, it's no wonder you're stressed out before your feet even hit the floor.

Do you have any idea what happens to your body when you have negative thoughts? Every thought we have, whether conscious or not, produces a physical response in the body. That means that stress, simply put, is the way your body reacts to your mind's thoughts. Whenever you feel anxious (a speech, a job interview, a tight deadline) or experience negative thoughts (I'm too fat; I'm too old; I can't handle this), your body swings into action, producing chemicals that gear you up to fight or flee. Hormones are released from your pituitary and adrenal glands. Your pulse speeds up.

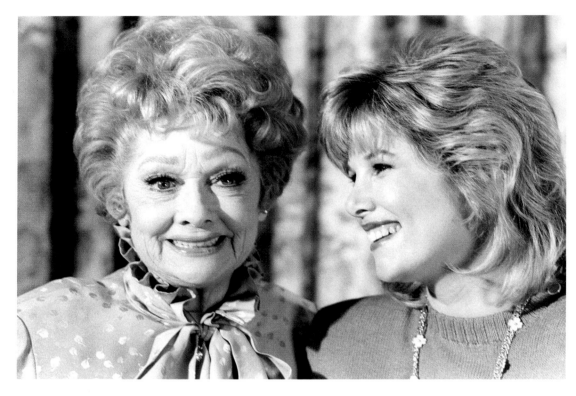

I always admired Lucille Ball, who never stopped taking chances and always found a way to make us laugh.

Your blood pressure rises. Your muscles tense. You start to perspire (to keep you cool under pressure). Your pupils dilate. Extra sugar and fat flow into your bloodstream (to give you quick energy). I was really amazed when I read about these physical responses in *Healing Mind, Healthy Woman* by Alice D. Domar and Henry Dreher, mainly because I recognized them. I have never considered myself a pessimist or a negative person, but no one is immune from the pitfalls of negative thinking. One of those phrases my mom taught me was to see the glass as half full rather than half empty. Yet self-doubt or a sense of being overwhelmed can make you feel negative at times, even if you're the most optimistic person. Self-doubt can even paralyze your ability to think clearly enough to make good decisions. Even my thirteen-year-old daughter, Lindsay, says that when she gets totally overwhelmed, her mind turns to mush. This kind of shutting down, or overreacting to a situation, usually ends up complicating the situation rather than resolving the problem.

We have become culturally conditioned to accept negative thinking as the norm. When I overhear people talking at work or on the street, most of the time they are complaining. Sadly, it's become the way we communicate, the way we get to know each other. We make friends by sharing our gripes instead of our enthusiasms. Sometimes we will have a valid reason for feeling negative about things. Maybe we are in a failing marriage, or we've had a disappointing relationship, or we're suffering from total overload from trying to be everything to everybody. Most of us can handle a few layers of stress simultaneously, but add six or seven layers and we begin to feel buried. If those layers escalate to nine? Hello, meltdown!

Negative thoughts are like emotional thieves who are on *your* payroll. You're the one who hired these thieves to rob you, and they come to steal your energy, your self-esteem, and your good days filled with joy. These rotten thieves cloud your ability to deal with crises and greatly limit your overall potential by preventing you from even trying new things. You have the choice to fire them. But it can't be done by suppressing or ignoring those feelings. You have to stop paying them—that is, you have to stop believing in them. If you let go of your negative thoughts, positive thoughts will start taking their place.

> *"One of the things I learned the hard way was it does not pay to get discouraged. Keeping busy and making optimism a way of life can restore your faith in yourself."*
> LUCILLE BALL

Psychologists such as Dr. Ellen McGrath say that negative thinking comes in several forms, but the following three are the key categories:

Personalization. You see yourself as the cause of something that you really weren't responsible for.

Magnification or minimization. You blow something out of proportion and make a big deal out of nothing, or inappropriately diminish the importance of a situation.

All-or-nothing thinking. A favorite among women, because with this kind of either/or thinking, we can feel like total failures if we're not totally perfect.

Don't know about you, but I am in touch with these classifications—up close and personal! It's normal to feel this way from time to time, but you just have to learn how to cope with life's ups and downs so they don't send you into a tailspin. You can overcome negative thinking patterns by learning to identify and understand your self-sabotaging behavior.

"My tormentor is myself left over from yesterday."
DEEPAK CHOPRA

I have learned to recognize when I'm being self-deprecating, but that doesn't mean that the negative thoughts simply evaporate. These days, when I'm being too hard on myself, I employ some really great methods I have learned to help me bring my mood back around. I call these my mood busters. One thing I find helpful when I am faced with a stressful situation is to remove myself from the scene. I take a walk or go for a drive. Sometimes I'll even take a long weekend away somewhere and really pamper myself with a massage and a facial or just sit on the beach doing nothing! Usually I find that a little time out helps me see things more clearly and handle them better. The old advice to "sleep on it" draws on the same reasoning. And it works! Miraculously, the solution to a problem often comes to us not when we concentrate most intently on it but when we have forgotten all about it—like when we're in the shower, too wet to write it down.

I have also found that music is a great mood buster for me. Feeling a little down? Put on some fun, funky, upbeat music and watch it turn your mood right around. Conversely, if you're feeling uptight and totally tense, try some mellow, relaxing music to bring you back to a calm, peaceful place. For even greater results, try singing out loud to your favorite compact disc. When I'm driving in my car, I'll sing my heart out. I have sung duets with Alanis Morissette, Sheryl Crow, M People, Celine Dion, and Gloria Estefan—and they don't even know it!

Like any red-blooded American girl, I find that going out for a day of shopping with a close friend is always a great way to bust my mood—though it might be a little more expensive than singing or taking a walk! I'm not suggesting that you go on a wild shopping spree, because that can only make things worse when those credit card bills appear. Plan a nice lunch with a friend you haven't seen for a while. Maybe get a manicure and pedicure—especially if you don't even need one! By the end of the day, I'm sure you'll feel a little better.

Finally, when I'm in a funk, I'll pick up the phone and reconnect with an old friend, someone I haven't spoken to for a while. It's always fun to catch up and reminisce about old times. And maybe you'll find an opportunity to help someone else with a problem, just by being a good listener. And you know what? You just might realize that helping someone else can make you feel better too. By helping others, I often learn something new or reinforce what I already know. That's reason enough to feel good about yourself.

We're Our Own Worst Critics

You hate the shape of your nose. Your hair's the wrong color. When you're alone, you study your flaws in the mirror, picking yourself completely apart. You wear baggy clothes to hide the shape of your body. If any of this sounds familiar, you may have a negative body image, like most American women. We are definitely our own worst critics. According to psychologist Dr. Ellen McGrath, "Research suggests that three out of four times, a woman's thoughts about her body are negative ones. For a number of women, there is nothing positive about their bodies."

Think about the comments you make to yourself over the course of just one morning. When you get dressed, check your makeup in the car mirror, or see your reflection in a store window, do you think nice things about your looks,

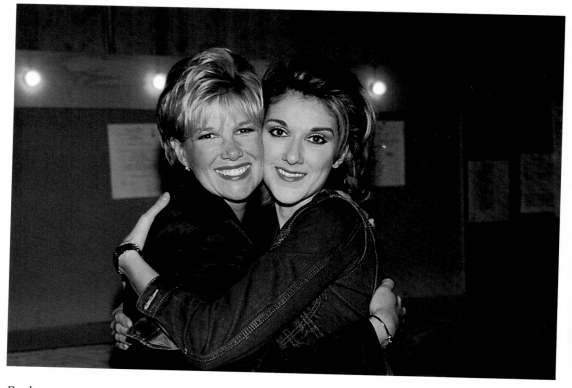

Backstage on tour with Celine Dion.

or are you critical? At least 75 percent of the time, we're very hard on ourselves. We say, "My thighs are too fat," "My skin is blotchy," or "I look terrible in this outfit." You would never treat a friend like that, so how come you do it to yourself?

But we all do it. Even Celine Dion. When I interviewed her for my *Behind Closed Doors* special, she told me when she looks in the mirror, she says to herself, "We'll fix that, we'll pluck this.... C'mon, honey, I want a smaller nose, I want bigger eyes, I want fuller lips, I want more boobs, I want—I mean, c'mon, I'm a normal girl, you know."

But Celine doesn't get too carried away with her wish list of changes. A lot of people were surprised to hear that when I traveled with her on the road, Celine would walk out of her hotel with no makeup and her hair not done. She

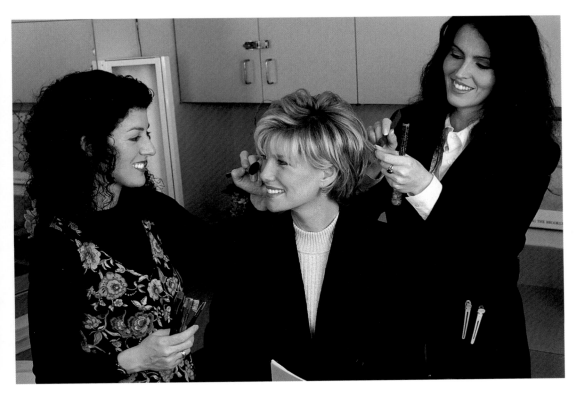

Makeup artist Michelle Cutler and hairstylist Kristin Barry help keep me looking my best.

was constantly meeting fans, who seemed to embrace her natural look. And at the concert hall where she's to perform, Celine does her entire rehearsal in a very casual mode, wearing a T-shirt, jeans, and no makeup. Celine's obvious comfort with herself is the reason people find her so endearing.

Women make themselves crazy by comparing themselves to an image they see in a magazine. The key word here is "image." I have been photographed for the magazines, so I know that what you see isn't always what you get. Once for a cover they even changed the color of my jacket from lavender to red, using the computer. What you're looking at on the pages of magazines is an image created by an industry solely to sell you a dress or a product. In fact, in my last *Behind Closed Doors* special, I did a

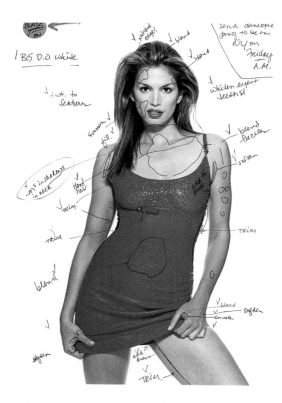

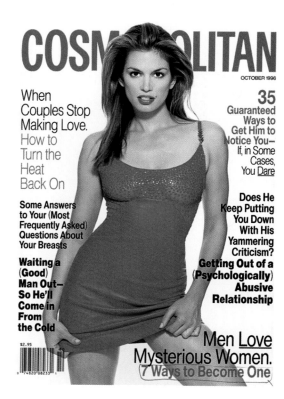

What you see isn't always what you get.

segment revealing the secrets used by the modeling industry to make those supermodels so super. You'd be amazed at the pinning and clamping that take place to make that slinky black dress fall so perfectly. Oh, and don't forget the duct tape under the breasts to make them a little perkier. A pinch here and a tuck there, and violà! But hold on to your brassiere...because even after that

photo is taken, the model can be altered to perfection. On my special we showed how a company called NEC used computer digitizing to alter a *Cosmopolitan* magazine cover. People were surprised to see that even a supermodel's perfect photogenic body undergoes retouching. They erased shadows under the model's eyes, removed wrinkles from her face and hands, and even shaved a few inches from the backs of her arms and thighs! So the next time you start to compare yourself to a magazine photo, realize that you might be unfairly setting yourself up by comparing yourself to an ideal that doesn't even exist.

Where does this negative self-image come from, anyway? It can start as early as childhood. My family was very supportive, but I remember hearing other parents make comments to their children such as "You'd be such a pretty girl if you lost a little weight." Maybe your brother teased you about your nose. Or you might have been told that people would think you were conceited if you liked your looks. Even if your parents had only positive things to say about you, maybe you heard your father put down other women or remark that your mother always seemed to be on a diet. Those kinds of statements send two messages: that a woman's job is to look good, and that it's appropriate for women to worry about measuring up.

Think about all of the time you wasted analyzing and agonizing over your appearance and your weight. Think of the fun experiences you've made yourself miss: "I can't go to my high school reunion unless I lose twenty pounds," or "I can't put a bathing suit on this body!"

Obviously, women would be a lot better off if they could redirect all of that energy into positive and productive thoughts.

Nonreactive Behavior

"Walk away from it until you're stronger. All your problems will be there when you get back, but you'll be better able to cope."
Lady Bird Johnson

I noticed that the more I started to change my inner self, the more I liked the results. So the better the results, the more I wanted to continue to grow and learn. It's like discovering a new toy that you just can't stop playing with.

The overflow effect has reached every area of my life. I speak my mind and I try to listen with an openness that I never knew before. Sometimes, especially as a parent of teenage girls, that openness is tested, and I mean really tested. I love an analogy that author Jon Kabat-Zinn used when I interviewed him for this book. He referred to children as our own live-in Zen masters. Their purpose and goal in life is to push all of our buttons and to constantly test us and see how we will react. He explained that it's not as if they are just trying to get a rise out of us—at least not all the time. It's that they are their own human beings and they have their own ideas about how they should be. Boy, do they ever! But if you're smart about reacting to those situations, a more compassionate, understanding, and calm response will bring you closer to your children, and you can use these interactions to do some work on yourself as well.

A few years ago I was introduced to the concept of nonreactive behavior. Sometime around New Year's Day of 1995 I decided to try to be less reactive to people and circumstances. Have you ever seen a young child fall down? There is always a moment of silence before the child reacts. If the parent rushes over and panics, inevitably the child starts to cry. But if the parent realizes that the child is fine and does not panic, usually the child pops right back up and goes on his merry way. For every action there must be a reaction, and usually it's how *we* react to something that determines the outcome.

Testing the Theory

Stress is the body's response to the mind's thoughts. Unless the body's built-in involuntary-response mechanism is triggered, you can choose how to react to any given situation. Nonreactive behavior is the practice of assessing a situation prior to formulating your response. It's rising above life's tough emotional challenges by remaining cool, calm, and collected. Once you make up your mind to practice nonreactive behavior, almost everything will be affected positively by your response.

Think of it this way: When children do something inappropriate, we as parents give them a time-out. Our hope is that they will think about what was wrong with their behavior and learn from their experience for next time. It's a forced period of reflection. Well, the same philosophy can hold true for us as adults. We can give ourselves a time-out and use the time to look at a situation before we react to it. Then, chances are, we will respond out of careful thought and consideration rather than pure emotion. A highly charged emotional response like shouting or throwing something is usually a regretted response. Give yourself a chance to think about the repercussions of your actions. Count to ten or take a break; then come back to discuss the situation calmly and rationally.

Though you may find that it is a constant challenge to practice nonreactive behavior, I assure you that it's worth it.

Last year I had what might be called the supreme test of nonreactive behavior. I came home after work to find my daughter Jamie in her bathroom with hot-pink foam bubbling atop her head. I looked at her and said, "Please tell me that the color on your head in no way resembles the color your hair will be." Jamie replied that it was *her* head and *her* hair. She also said that it was unrealistic for me to expect her always to have it a normal color in the 1990s. It was her right to choose! All I know is: this kid should become a lawyer.

I felt myself starting to say those words I swore I would never say as a parent. You know the ones I'm talking about. Your parents said them to you, too: "Well, this is my house and I make the rules, and so long as you live in my house you'll live by my rules!" I couldn't

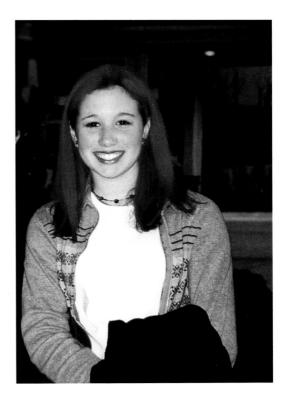

Jamie at age fifteen... pretty in pink.

believe those words were coming from my lips! Obviously they had been planted there years before, and they just popped right out. So I decided to take a time-out. I really thought about all the teenage battles a parent might have to face in today's world. From that perspective, pink hair seemed pretty far down that list. Did I love the color? Well, actually, it was kind of a pretty pink. Was I happy that my daughter would be running around with pink hair? Well, no, but it could have been worse. She could have shaved her boyfriend's initials into her scalp.

So when she came to dinner that night with her now blown-dry hot-pink hair, I gave her absolutely no reaction. As she sat at the dinner table that night, there was an awkward moment of silence, and then I calmly said, "It's not the pink hair that bothers me as much as the fact that you didn't ask me first." To which my young lawyer-to-be replied, "But if I had asked you, you would have just said no." Okay, I could see that this was a big test, so I dropped the subject and just passed her the pasta.

My nonreaction surprised and maybe even disappointed her. I mean why does a teenager dye her hair hot pink in the first place, if not to get a reaction? Now, I will say that it was a bit easier for me to assume this new nonreactive stance, as opposed to donning my battle gear, since I knew this would be a short-lived expression of her identity. In a few months the horse show season would gear up again, and that's a very traditional sport; hot-pink hair would not go over big in the show ring. I also knew Jamie well enough to know her competitive spirit wouldn't allow her to risk it with the judges. Eventually it would have to be dyed back to a color that grows on a head naturally. There was no need to turn this battle into a war that could have cut off our communication.

I guess the moral of this story is to pick your battles. Teenagers will be teenagers, and they will test your patience. You don't have to like everything that your children do, but you might have to accept some things that you weren't prepared for. You certainly aren't going to love your kids any less for dyeing their hair, and you have to give them enough freedom to make their own choices. Maybe they'll discover that it wasn't "them" to have pink hair. If you insist on making every decision for them, then you also stand in the way of their development. That's not to say we shouldn't set boundaries as parents, because we should, but we also need to understand the consequences of our reactions to our children's behavior.

Remember, the key to staying nonreactive is to take that step back and pick a response that will elicit the best reaction from everyone.

Something else besides teenagers can try my patience and test my ability to be nonreactive. I'll give you a hint. It's another word that begins with a *T*. . . . Can you say "tabloid"?

One of the unfortunate consequences of being a celebrity is having the press constantly writing about my personal life. They write about men I have dated, men I have stopped dating, and even about men I have never dated: "Joan Lunden Falls for L.L. Cool J at Party in Hollywood!" Huh? I guess it would have been a lot more boring to write "Joan Lunden Helps Daughter Lindsay Do Homework in Connecticut!" According to the press I have figured out a way to be on both coasts at the same time.

Another of my family's favorite tabloid headlines was that I was going to marry Shaquille O'Neil. Now that's what I call "hoop dreams"! I said a few years ago that my New Year's resolution was to start having half as much fun as the tabloids say I do. But when they have me dancing on tables, and jumping from the arms of one young hunk to another, they're making it awfully hard to keep up!

In the grand prize–winning headline to date one of the tabloids listed me as one of the ten most scandalous women in America. I had the pleasure of reading that one night while I was sitting around the house with my daughters watching *Home Improvement.* Their response was, "If you're one of the most scandalous women in America, Mom, then this must be a pretty boring country!"

Needless to say, all of this focus on my love life makes it incredibly difficult to have a private life. It also impedes the ability to let a relationship develop normally. If I reacted to every article, every tabloid story, and every mention I get on a weekly basis, I could spend a lot of time being annoyed. Who needs that? You know the old saying, "Like water off a duck's back"? Most of the time I try to keep my sense of humor and get a pretty good laugh out of the b.s. that is written. As for the other stories, the more hurtful ones, so long as they don't target my children I must take the attitude that I will let go and rise above them. This is called *really* taking the higher road!

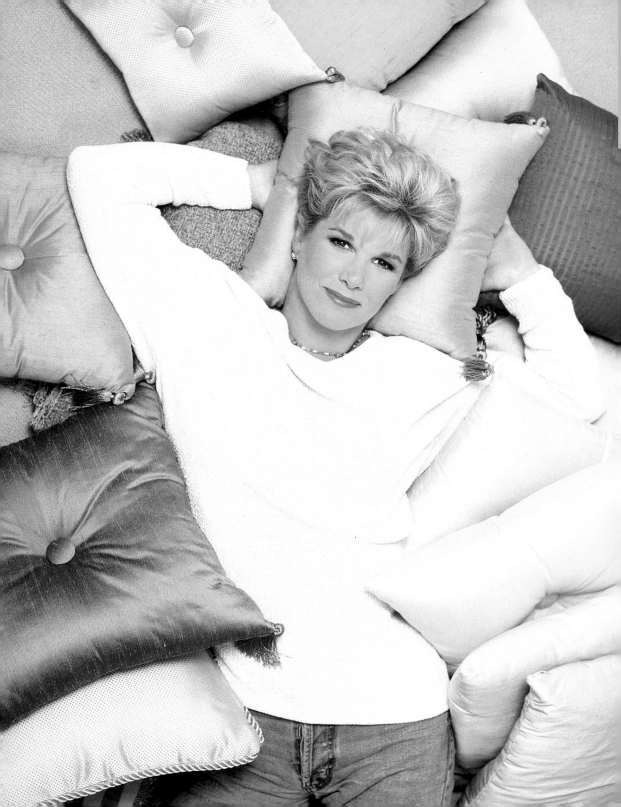

5 Relaxation and De-Stressing Techniques

It is possible to access an inner refuge from even the most traumatic event. Eliciting the relaxation response offers that port in the storm.

—DR. ALICE DOMAR

True relaxation—the kind that relieves you of all of your daily pressures, stresses, and obligations—isn't easy. First of all, most of us don't make nearly as much time as we should to slow down and smell the roses. It has taken me years to discover that I can "turn it off," even if I only have ten minutes. I think most of us think of relaxation as a luxury, like something we can only do on vacation, so it is usually the first thing to go when our schedule gets full.

For me, the best way to combat the unwanted and unneeded side effects that come with living a hectic life was to gain a better understanding of the concept of meditation. I'm the kind of person who gets bogged down in that mind chatter I mentioned earlier. It happens as I go to sleep at night, even as I'm trying to practice positive thinking. I finally fall into bed after another long day, and my mind fills with thoughts and ideas. My heart races, and I start to panic because I'm not falling asleep. So I toss and turn, my mind chattering away—sleep, *sleep!* I keep looking at the clock and before I know it, it's time to get up! Ugh! Another sleepless night! Sound like anyone you know?

Many of your so-called relaxing activities may actually add more tension and stress to your already crazy life. Do you drink a cup (or a pot) of coffee during high-tension times of the day? How about right before you go to sleep? What about smoking, drinking, or eating? Caffeine, alcohol, and any other stimulant can really strain your system, especially if you're totally stressed out. Even watching television is thought by some experts to cause nervous tension, as

was documented in *The U.C. Berkeley Wellness Encyclopedia,* based on studies performed at the university (although they say that morning shows were not included in this research!). Apparently the high-frequency TV images can interfere with brain-wave patterns.

Making the time to practice relaxation and de-stressing techniques is essential to establishing wellness in your life. It requires discipline, but the results are remarkable. You'll have more energy, better sleep, more focus and concentration, and an overall calmness to your approach in life. It's all about making yourself a priority. Now, isn't that incentive enough to read on?

Simple Relaxation Techniques

Relaxation techniques nourish you on a deep plane so that you can achieve a higher level of mind-body awareness. One of the simplest techniques is called progressive relaxation. Believe it or not, I was first turned on to this technique by my dentist, Dr. Ralph Kranin. Being slightly dental phobic, I need this technique just to get through a general teeth cleaning. You'll find it's a great way to achieve total calmness and serenity. The object is to relax your entire body. Begin by repeating slowly and softly the following four words: *calm...peaceful... tranquil...relaxed...*Imagine all of the stress and anxiety in your body being released through this exercise. Get a picture of that unwanted stress leaving your body, progressing up through your body, first through your toes, then your feet, ankles, calves, knees, thighs, butt, abdomen, lower back, chest, shoulders, arms, wrists, hands, fingers, neck, face, and head. By the time you get to your scalp, you ought to be completely relaxed. I usually start to fall asleep somewhere around the hips, but if you can make it farther than that, hey, go for it! Really focus on each body part and on the idea of letting that stress go, but don't forget to repeat those four words: *calm...peaceful...tranquil... relaxed...*There are a lot of audiotapes available at most bookstores that utilize this technique.

Another excellent relaxation technique is a simple visualization exercise. I remember the early days when I first started working out with fitness expert Barbara Brandt. She tried so hard to impress upon me the importance of stretching and relaxation. This was a challenge for her, since at the time I only cared about getting on the treadmill and burning calories. After a workout we would sit on the floor and stretch. Barbara would guide me through a series of breathing and visualization exercises that helped me relax and get a better stretch. She would have me close my eyes and visualize the muscle that I was stretching. She said to see the muscle like lots of pieces of spaghetti intertwined. As I stretched, I was to imagine the muscle slowly unraveling. This kind of total concentration on relaxing the muscle makes it virtually impossible to tighten or contract the muscle at the same time. Your brain can't accommodate two opposing forces simultaneously. This must be what "mind over matter" means! This process really helped my flexibility.

Another visualization exercise Barbara taught me focused on breathing. She guided me through a series of breathing exercises, asking me to close my eyes and see a beautiful color as I inhaled. As I exhaled I was to see the

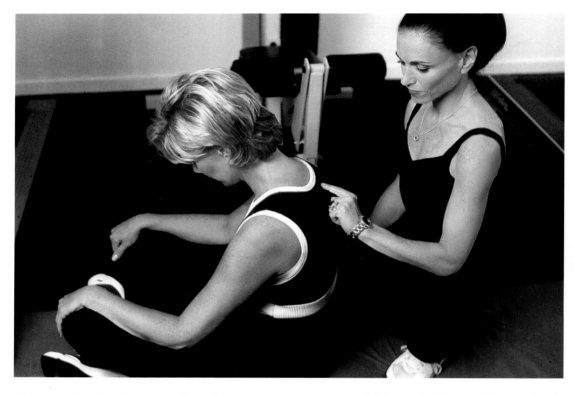

Fitness trainer Barbara Brandt teaching me
relaxation through visualization.

color flowing through my muscles, intensifying in color, taking the tension right out of my body. It took some practice, but I got it, and it definitely helped me to relax and mellow out after a workout.

If all of this seems just a little too far out there to start with, try another of Barbara's techniques. I like to use it with my kids, and I'll bet if you think back, your mom and dad probably did this with you when you were a child. Barbara would have me sit on the floor and close my eyes. Then she would very very gently draw letters on my back. I was to concentrate on nothing but feeling each line on my skin, and guessing which letter was being drawn. It sounds very simple, but it takes concentration and is an easy introduction to how visualization can help you relax.

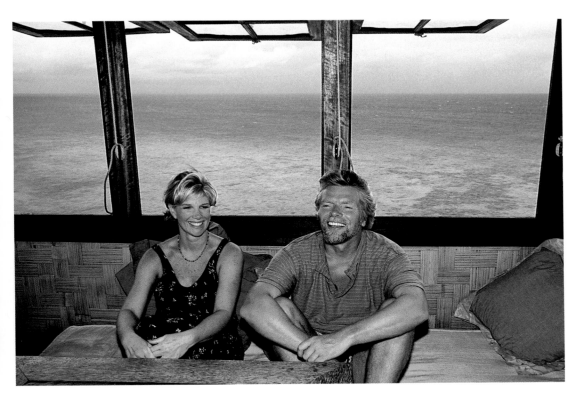

Creating Your Own Quiet Space

High above the blue Caribbean, Richard Branson shows me around his quiet space, Bali H'ai.

How do *you* unwind after a crazy, hectic day? Do you find it difficult to escape all of the demands of kids, your mate, your boss, or anything else that may be part of your life? Everyone can benefit from finding some time alone for herself. It's not easy, but you must essentially make an appointment with yourself. After you spend some time alone, even if it's just a half hour, you will find that your mind is clearer and that your thoughts are purer. It took me years to truly understand the importance of taking time alone with myself.

Whether you practice a form of meditation, learn some easy breathing exer-

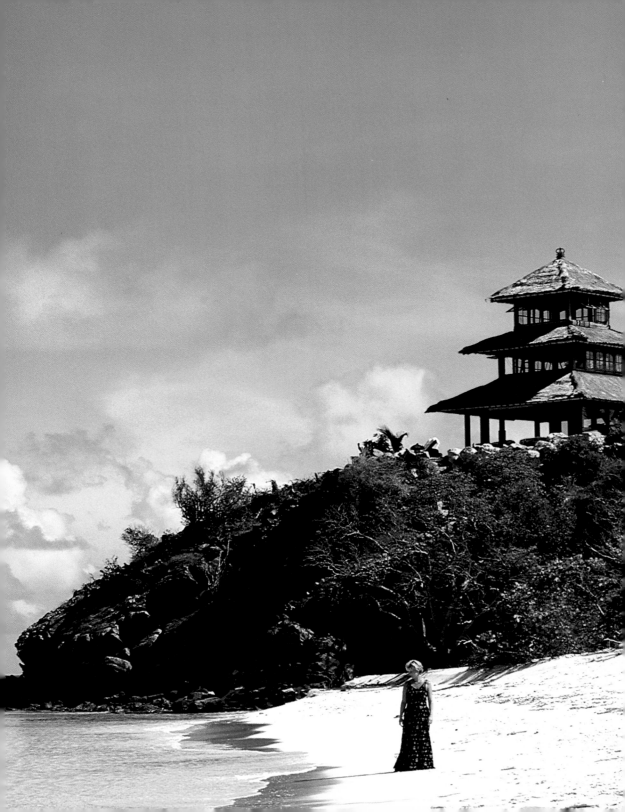

cises to let go of that mind chatter, or simply practice a relaxation exercise, it's much more effective if you have a designated space that is meant for that purpose, allowing you to escape those daily stresses. I have an area in my home that I have dedicated to the art of practicing meditation. However, a quiet place can be found anywhere, anytime. It's more of an attitude and a spiritual outlook than an actual physical space.

Some people take this concept to an extreme. While shooting my fourth *Behind Closed Doors* prime-time special, I visited Necker Island in the Caribbean. Necker Island is a private island owned by billionaire Richard Branson. As if owning your own island isn't enough, I was fascinated to learn that he'd had two Balinese meditation temples transported to this "fantasy island." Piece by piece they were dismantled on the island of Bali and transported by ship along with six Balinese craftsmen who fully reconstructed the structures on the island. When asked why he didn't just build

Bali H'ai, the private retreat on Necker Island, Richard Branson's Caribbean getaway.

replicas, Richard replied that the feeling would never be the same. Sitting on the top floor of his three-tiered temple, I could feel the centuries of peacefulness and serenity. As I perched atop this extraordinary structure, I truly had a sense of that feeling he was talking about.

As a man who runs megacompanies such as Virgin Atlantic Airlines, Virgin Cola, and Virgin Music, Richard Branson understands the demands of a hectic lifestyle and knows the importance of getting away and relaxing. He explained his philosophy to me:

In life you've got to play hard as well as work hard to get the right balance. I'm lucky I'm able to do that. Last night I was sitting outside with my children. Every three minutes a shooting star came right over our heads. You know there are a lot of kids who will never experience lying back, seeing this wonderful clear sky, and the marvels of what goes on above us.

Needless to say, you don't need your own private island or Balinese temple to find your own peacefulness and serenity. Goldie Hawn recently spoke to me on *Good Morning America* about the importance of taking time to nurture oneself. She said that she has her quiet place, a room in her home in which she meditates.

Goldie created this room to house her spirit. She sits surrounded by talismans—crystals and prayer beads and Buddhas—that she says stimulate her "energy and point of view and sense of groundedness in terms of belonging to the universe." Goldie is very committed to the pursuit of her spiritual ideals. "His Holiness the Dalai Lama recently gave me a mantra, which I love," says Hawn, who has been meditating for years. She says, "The more evolved you are in terms of who you are in relation to the big picture, the more enlightened you become as to where you want your life to go. The bottom line is, this is your life."

For Oprah Winfrey, quiet space is in the elevator that takes her twelve stories down to the studio where she tapes her show. In the August 1996 *Redbook,* she says:

Here I try to center myself to only put out good. You know you're going to be speaking to millions of people, so you want anything that you say or do to be done for the good of everybody who's going to hear you. My prayer to God every morning on my knees is that the power that is in the universe should use my life as a vessel or a vehicle for its work. Prayer. That is the central thing for me.

A space to "peace out" and let go can be anywhere so long as it provides enough privacy and stillness to allow you to relax.

When I was married, way before I knew anything about meditation or the need for creating my own space, I ironically found one anyway. The only place in my house that at that moment in my life offered me private space was what many people think of as the "thinker's spot." Okay, you guessed it—my bathroom! So it wasn't a Balinese temple (see, I told you don't need your own temple!), but it was a place where I could take time for myself. Of course, back then, I probably used this time and place as a means of escape, avoiding the obvious anguish of a crumbling marriage, an incredibly overloaded schedule, and all of the demands I felt were placed on me at the time. Today, rather than running away from all of the pressures, I manage them better by taking time alone and stepping back to look at my life. From a fresh perspective, you will always have a greater ability to guide your own path.

I now reserve my bathroom for showering, blowing my hair dry, and putting on my makeup. I take my quiet moments in a corner of my bedroom. I chose this spot for a reason. My home is in the middle of a forest, and the walls of my bedroom are all windows, allowing me to look out into the woods and feel that I am one with nature. The mood is immediately peaceful and serene, and I appreciate how lucky I am to have this at my doorstep. I sit between my sofa and glass coffee table, which is covered with candles that I light during these moments. As I slip into my quiet spot, I always put on some tranquil music. I enjoy "The Mariner" by new age musician Tony O'Connor, available through the Natural Wonders stores. It incorporates the sounds of the ocean, nature, and the Pan flute, which I love. I also like to listen to Enigma.

While I designated this space for myself several years ago, it is only in recent years that I have actually started to use it. The fact is, I was intimidated by the thought of spending time alone with myself. I was also uncomfortable with the idea of slowing down, because my norm is to go a million miles an hour.

Interestingly, the more I have used my quiet space, the more rewards I feel I gain from it. It's kind of like a muscle that is strengthened by use. Today I find it most beneficial in helping me sink into deep relaxation at night and allowing me to go to sleep more easily. It also gives me a place to let go of anger and stress and to put things into perspective. It lets me see mole hills as mole hills and not turn them into mountains. In the end, it fills me with gratitude for all that I have. It sends me back to my family, co-workers, and friends with a renewed appreciation of them, and everyone around me then reaps the benefits of that time as well.

Breathing

If I had to say that there was a miracle cure for almost every problem in life, I would have to choose breathing. This

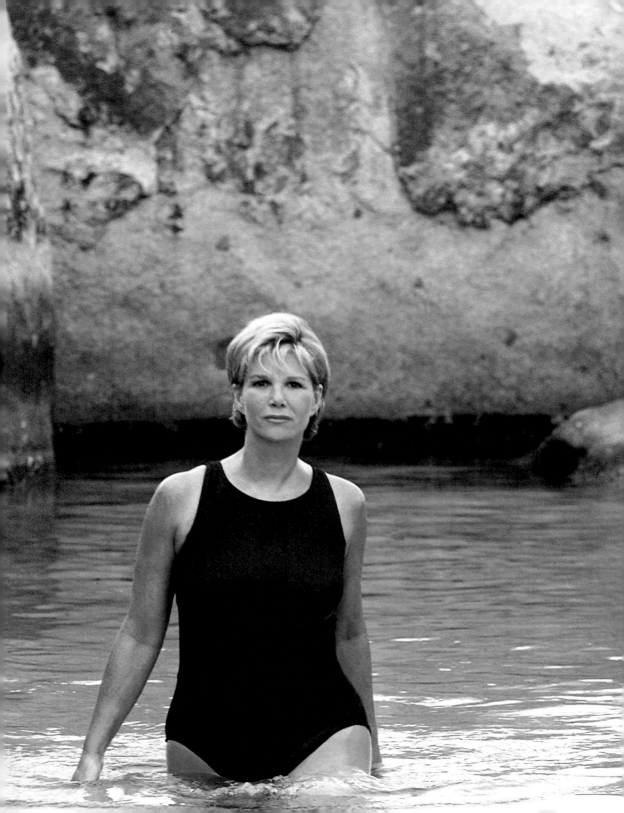

discovery came as such a revelation for me, since it's something that we all take for granted. Most of us don't realize we can use relaxed breathing to help control our emotions, reduce stress, quiet our body, and focus on our thoughts—all things that we want to cultivate and weave throughout every aspect of our lives. If you are tense and stressed, breathing can return your body to a normal level. If you are facing an important decision, stop and breathe. Whenever you have a question in your mind about what to do next or how to do it, just breathe. Breathing is the most crucial element of strong emotional and spiritual health. How you feel shows in the way you breathe.

I never realized that tension and stress had an impact on breathing. Anxiety creates shallow, ineffective breathing, and I discovered that in stressful situations I would actually hold my breath. When I'm working out, my trainer Pat Manocchia has to constantly remind me to breathe, a crucial part of keeping exercise effective. My riding instructor,

Learning good breathing techniques helps me relax and enjoy everything I do to the fullest.

Kip Rosenthal, says that every time I enter a competition, I hold my breath as I navigate the entire course. I don't need to tell you that this is not a great idea. I can always hear Kip yelling from the sidelines, "Joan...*breathe!*"

Breathing is the foundation of relaxation techniques and meditation. Try this simple exercise: Take a deep breath through your nostrils, and send this breath first into your lower chest, and then all the way down to your belly. Feel the breath as it moves through your body. Now slowly release this breath, again almost watching it as it moves up and out. Count as you inhale, and try to match the length of the exhalation. Do this three or four times, concentrating on keeping your breathing even and slow.

As you repeat this process, you will begin to feel your body start relaxing and almost slow down to match the pace of your breathing. With your total concentration on this slow calm breathing, your muscles will loosen and your mind will clear. You can't concentrate on other things if you're totally concentrating on your breathing.

This is all it takes to begin the process

of deep, healthy breathing. (Of course, anyone who has ever taken voice or singing lessons knows the importance of this deep diaphragm breathing. That's how opera singers can hold those notes so long.) Practice your breathing regularly—driving to work in the morning, cooking dinner, and before you go to sleep. With this calming technique perfected, you'll be able to call upon it in times of stress and better able to handle difficult situations.

It is important to pay attention as you practice your breathing. Let each inhalation empower you, and let go of tension and stress on each exhalation. The rhythm of your breathing sets a calmer pace for your mind and spirit. Clear your mind, if only momentarily, and focus on the sensation of your breathing. Try not to let outside distractions interfere with the process, and definitely try to keep your mind chatter to a minimum and eventually at zero. The ultimate goal is to sharpen your ability to concentrate, tap into a calmer and more stable state of being, and be better able to make clearer decisions. In Chapter 6 I'll talk about breathing being an integral part of meditation.

Bath Rituals

At the end of a long day, one of my favorite things to do is to run a hot bath, light my many aromatic candles, and immerse myself in the tub. Something about the sensation of feeling weightless in the water helps the tension and stress of a rigorous day evaporate. I find that there is no place like the bath to close my eyes and reflect. I think about the past days, and I make plans for the future. I use this peaceful time to listen to my inner voice and let it help guide my actions. I try to keep my focus on the positive aspects of all situations I am facing, making this bath time an uplifting ritual.

Try adding some aromatic essential oils to your bath, like lavender, which has a calming quality. Its fragrance is thought to help balance the mind, body, and spirit. Eucalyptus is often cited as an expectorant, easing respiratory ailments, and is even said to increase concentration. Chamomile (just like chamomile tea) is often noted for relieving tension and muscle tightness and for its calming effects. Aromatic bath crystals are also great for therapy, especially after a hard

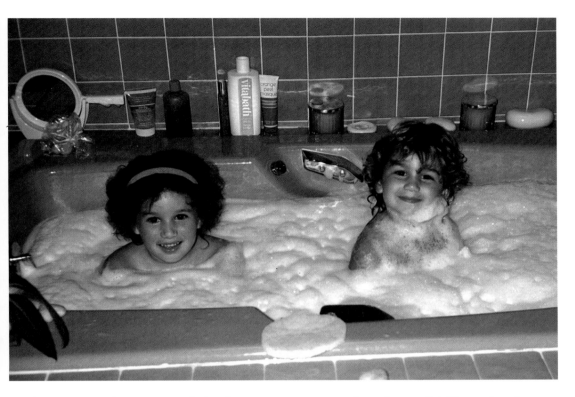

Jamie and Lindsay will kill me when they see this picture!

workout to soothe tense and tired muscles. You can even use plain old Epsom salts. Sometimes I'll just make a wonderful bubble bath and let the bubbles soak up any anxiety from my day. Of course, I know through years of research which bubble bath makes the best bubbles, having given my girls millions of baths over their lifetime. While Mr. Bubble builds bountiful bubbles, I do believe that it was a bottle of Winnie-the-Pooh bubble bath that produced the sea of bubbles for

Jamie and Lindsay when they were six and three.

Some soothing music is also a nice touch for your bath ritual, though sometimes I really just enjoy the serene atmosphere of just soaking in silence. I like to light candles while bathing and surround myself with their flickering light. The softness of their flames really helps set a

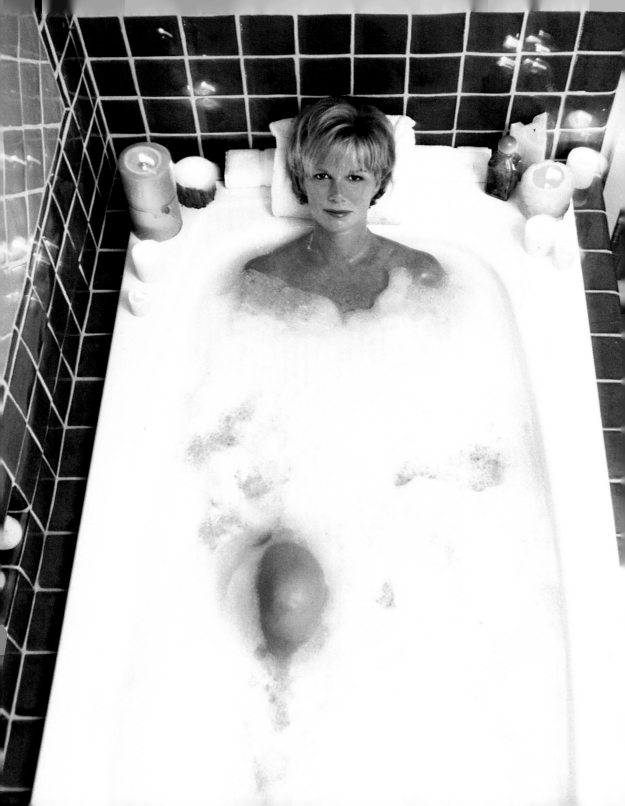

calm and relaxing mood, inducing an openness in my mind, body, and spirit. Surrounding yourself with this white light creates the feeling of a safe environment, and it makes me feel as though I have lit a path to my soul.

The most important part of your bath ritual is that you are taking this time to just do something nice for yourself. Give yourself a facial mask, indulge in some pretty handmade soaps, find a good book to read, or simply do nothing. However you decide to spend that time in the tub, make it special. You deserve it.

They say that water is the essence of and symbol of life. Our bodies are two-thirds water, as is the earth. Immersing yourself in water becomes a ritual of renewal and an affirmation of your life. Participating in an activity that helps us reconnect with ourselves is what a ritual is really all about. There is no discomfort in my life that a bath can't help soothe, even just a bit. *Ahhhh!* Now, don't you feel better already?

Taking a bath is one of the best gifts you can give yourself—as long as your kids let you share their bubble bath.

Massage

Most people think of massage as an extravagance. Maybe you'll treat yourself to a massage while on vacation or on that rare occasion when you're in the mood to pamper yourself. Whether this describes your massage history or not, I'm happy to report to you that massage is now considered by many experts to have tremendous psychological, physical, and emotional health benefits. In fact, after relaxation techniques and chiropractic therapy, massage is now the third most prevalent type of alternative medical treatment sought by American adults. Massage can reduce pain, ease tension, reduce anxiety and stress, and stimulate endorphins, the "feel good" chemicals in the brain. America is the only developed country where massage therapy is not yet an officially approved method of health care, though some insurance companies are starting to cover massage therapy. And if that still doesn't make massage mainstream enough for you, at the 1996 Summer Olympic Games, for the first time ever, the official Olympic medical services team included 120 massage therapists, who worked side by side with orthopedists, cardiologists, and other sports medicine professionals.

Massage may also boost the body's immune system. Researchers at the Medical College of Ohio in Toledo found that AIDS patients who received forty-five-minute massages once a week had lower levels of stress hormones and more so-called killer cells that attack tumors. Although the research wasn't conclusive about whether this increase in killer cells can actually prevent illness, it was clear that massage therapy did improve the patients' emotional state.

Clinical psychologist Robert Jamison of the Brigham and Women's Hospital Pain Management Center in Boston says, "If people believe something will help them get better, it often does. The body tends to follow the mind." If you think about it, what's the first thing you do when you stub your toe or bump your head? You rub the sore spot to alleviate the pain, right? Well, massage works the same way. By applying pressure, massage seems to close down the pain signals to the brain.

Massage is especially important for those of us who exercise a lot. It helps the body get rid of lactic acid, which is the stuff that makes muscles ache after a workout. Combining massage with a stretching and strength training program can even improve your posture and relieve lower back strain.

So now that we know that massage isn't just a selfish indulgence, how do you decide what kind of massage is right for you? There are four major types, each with its own benefits:

Swedish Massage. The most common form of massage, it is used to promote relaxation and circulation. It involves long strokes and kneading on bare skin, usually using massage oil or powder to reduce friction.

Shiatsu. Also known as acupressure, this is an Asian method that focuses on pressure points. Massage therapists use their hands, their elbows, and sometimes even their feet to apply the pressure. It's an effective method, though it may seem awkward or even painful to you at first if you've never tried massage.

Neuromuscular Massage. This deep-tissue massage is similar to Swedish but uses more pressure and a stronger touch to get deeper into those extra tight muscles.

Sports Massage. This combines a range of techniques to help athletes relax before workouts, games, or events. It also helps prevent soreness and promotes recovery after physical exercise.

There are other massage methods, like reflexology (similar to Shiatsu, but focusing on pressure points on the feet and hands) and aromatherapy. Massage therapists may use other names for these methods, based on where they received their training, but the procedure will for the most part be the same. Often the therapist will light candles and play restful music to create a relaxing environment.

Massage is something that I find the time to enjoy. Its short-term benefits are helpful in reducing stress, muscle soreness, and overall anxiety in my everyday life. Even if you don't have the time to get massaged on a regular basis, in larger cities, the Great American Back Rub stores seem to be opening up faster than Blockbuster Video these days. These storefront massage centers offer an inexpensive ten-minute quick-fix by qualified therapists, and even the busiest people can find ten minutes to relax.

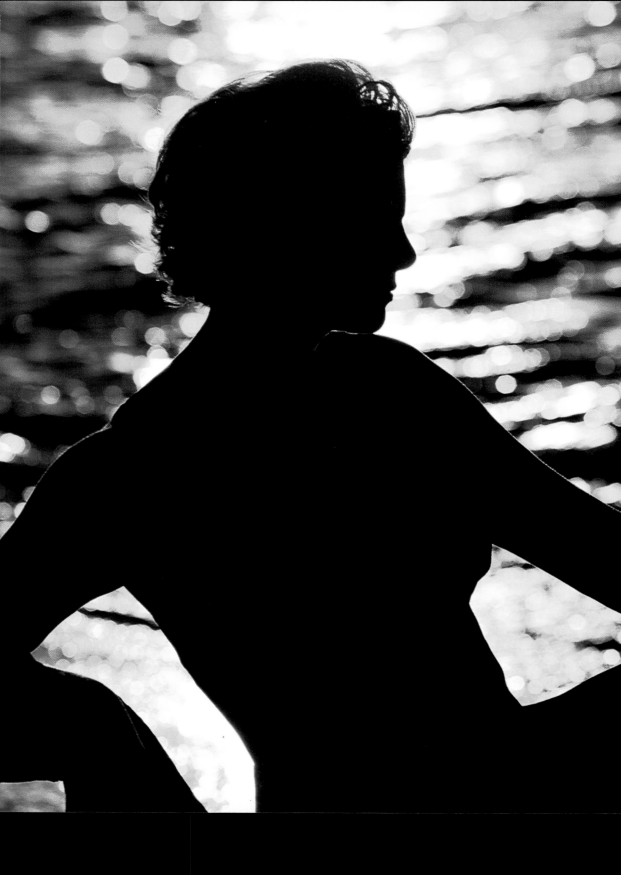

6 How Meditation Makes Your Life Better

Meditation is not an evasion,
it is a serene encounter with reality.

—ZEN MASTER THICH NHAT HANH

I am not an expert on meditation, but I have done a lot of reading on the subject and I practice the art regularly. The best definition I have ever read of what meditation is, and even what it is not, is by Jon Kabat-Zinn. In his book, *Wherever You Go, There You Are,* he says,

> When we speak of meditation, it is important for you to know that this is not some weird cryptic activity, as our popular culture might have it. It does not involve becoming some

kind of zombie, vegetable, self-absorbed narcissist, navel gazer, space cadet, cultist, devotee, mystic, or Eastern philosopher. It is a commonly held view that meditation is a way to shut off the pressures of the world or of your own mind, but this is not an accurate impression. Meditation is neither shutting things out nor off. It is seeing things clearly, and deliberately positioning yourself differently in relationship to them.

Meditation has gone pretty mainstream these days. According to Deepak Chopra, well-known author of several books, including *Ageless Body, Timeless Mind,* now that meditation has entered mainstream Western culture, researchers have finally applied scientific measurements to this subjective experience. It's been discovered that people who meditate function more efficiently psychologically. Deepak Chopra goes on to say that many of the physiological effects of stress that speed up the aging process are slowed and even, some experts believe, reversed through the process of meditation. One of the most fascinating aspects of this research, which has been ongoing for over

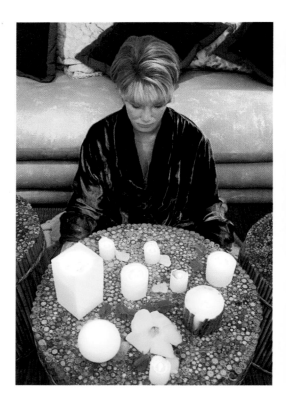

Looking inside.

two decades now, is that long-term meditators can have bodies that are physiologically comparable to typical bodies that are five to twelve years younger.

In fact it's quite well known that many professional athletes and sports teams including the Chicago Bulls use meditation as part of their training. One of the major results of meditation is a calming of the mind and a deeper level of relaxation. Meditation eases tension, and actually helps you become more accepting of others and, maybe more important, accepting of yourself. Meditation teaches you how to be your own best friend.

When you first begin to meditate, you should not expect too much too soon. The first day you start studying a foreign language you don't expect to speak it, right? I remember the first time I tried meditation. I was so scared that I wouldn't be able to do it. I really didn't know what to expect at first. Not only that, but since I live in a constant state of sleep deprivation, I was actually afraid that I might fall asleep. But the promise of learning how to take that look inward that I had heard so much about far outweighed my fear of not knowing what I was doing.

My friend Scot Evans first introduced me to the the idea of meditation. It took me a few years of talking about it to finally be ready. To make me more comfortable with this experience, he put together a meditation session with some of my closest friends. Over the past two and a half years he's walked hand in hand with me along this spiritual path I have chosen. He has witnessed some of the changes in me along the way.

Meditation helps Joan learn how to look inside for the answers rather than depend on outside forces and influences. Many women have been taught to depend on others for guidance. But self-trust is the first secret of personal success and empowerment. And this can be attained through meditation.

Joan has developed the confidence to be able to draw the best to and from herself, and she has become strengthened with her new voice.

She made a choice during these last few years to surround herself with people who have positive energy, and it has rubbed off on her. Joan has really felt this motivation, and it has shown up in her daily life. One way it comes through is on GMA. Joan is clearly the best she has ever been, not only on television but in her daily activities. Joan is also able to take this positive energy and share it with the people around her. Therefore, everyone around Joan now reaps the benefits of her positive energy.

As I sat there that first night, I was guided on a gentle journey through relaxation techniques that included deep methodical breathing and basic visualization skills. I realized that meditation is simply a way to disentangle ourselves from the clutter and chatter of our minds. Asian philosophers contend that meditation creates a balance and a flow of energy through the body. All I know is that I felt totally exhilarated by this experience, energized, and yet much more peaceful than when we started.

You'll need discipline and practice to achieve the full benefits of meditation. When you meditate, you want to find a comfortable position. Sit against something that supports your back. Sit as erect as possible while remaining relaxed and comfortable. Finding that steadying posture becomes essential as you practice meditation, so your breath will flow easily throughout the body. It suggests that you sit crossed-legged, but only if that's comfortable for you. If you choose to sit in a chair, your feet should be flat on the floor. (You can put a pillow behind your back if you need to sit more forward in the chair.) Assume the same position each time you meditate, so that you automatically associate it with that peaceful, calm state of mind. Though you don't have to close your eyes, it will probably help when you begin to learn.

If you choose to meditate with your eyes open be sure to focus on one spot. Allow yourself to focus on your breathing. As I said in Chapter 5, breathing is essential to all that we do, but it also has a natural calming effect, making it easier to reap the benefits of meditation. Don't just hear your breath; feel it. Try not to alter the pattern, but become aware of it. Inhale through the nostrils, exhale through the mouth. Take long, deep, slow breaths. Feel the air streaming in as you inhale, and visualize it flowing out of your body as you exhale. As you focus on your breathing, other thoughts will keep popping into your head. That's fine. They will come and then will go. Keep your focus on your breath until that chattering of your mind stops.

I'm sure you've heard that some people use a mantra—a word or phrase—when they meditate. This is another focusing tool used in meditation; it requires you to concentrate on nothing else but that mantra. You can use any word or short sentence that has meaning for you. Repeat your mantra either quietly out loud or to yourself, over and over, using it to clear your head of any other thoughts that may cloud your mind while meditating. You can also repeat the mantra in synch with the rhythm of your breathing. Meditation does not require using a mantra for it to be effective. In fact, you don't need anything except yourself and a few quiet moments. You can take it anywhere you go, because it is within you.

Be patient with meditation. After a few weeks you should find that you are calmer and more relaxed. You might be surprised at how energized you feel, too. As with any exercise, the results are not immediate, but they can be long-term if you keep up the workouts.

And speaking of workouts, meditation can even be used while you're working out, making it an active or moving meditation. You can even do a walking meditation while strolling through a park on your lunch break. Focus on your movements and your breathing. The more relaxed you are while exercising, the more efficiently you build muscle. For example, fitness expert Kathy Kaehler says that grimacing while running makes you clench your jaw, which tightens your muscles and hampers your breathing. She suggests smiling, which has an opposite effect.

Over time and with much practice, I have started to learn how to better put things into perspective, and I believe meditation has had a key role in this development. It has become easier to analyze and prioritize the events of my day, my week, and my upcoming year. Meditation has become a soothing silence and stillness in my life, and the benefits are as important to me as the physical benefits of exercise.

Perhaps my greatest revelation about meditation is that it has given me the ability to live for today and to enjoy each moment. I used to always spend my todays making my plans for my tomorrows. Meditation provides me with the ability to embrace each moment.

Within you there is a stillness and
sanctuary to which you can retreat
at any time and be yourself.
This sanctuary is a simple awareness
of comfort, which can't be violated
by the turmoil of events.
This place feels no trauma and
stores no hurt. It is the healing mental
* space*
that one seeks to find
in meditation.

—HERMANN HESSE

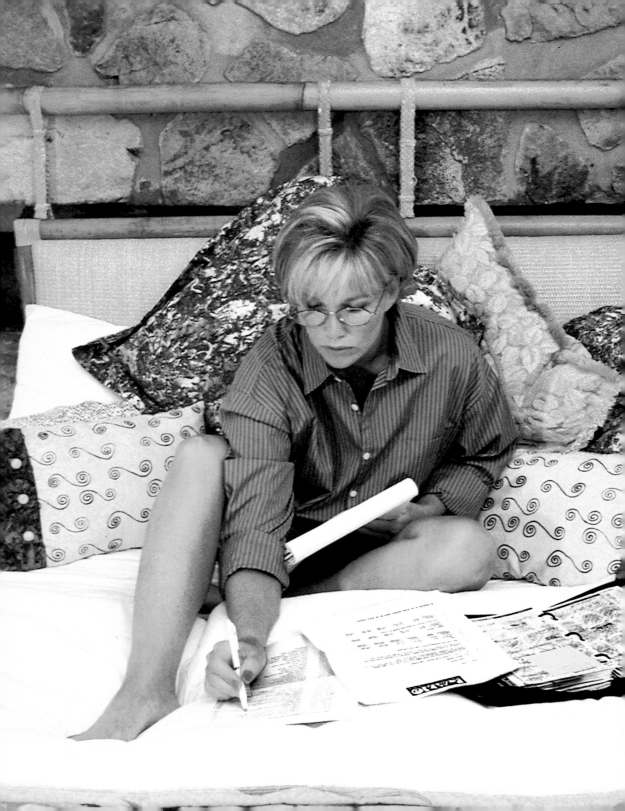

7 Dealing with Change

My friends laugh at me for being so organized, but it's one way I can better deal with change.

—JOAN LUNDEN

Life in every aspect is ever-changing, unpredictable, and uncontrollable by most standards. Our ability to deal with all of the unknowns—change, in particular—will really determine the outcome of our journey.

Dealing productively with change is recognizing the possibilities for hearing something in a new way or for seeing that you don't have to react in the way you always have. You have an enormous amount of control over your emotions—you can make a conscious decision to be calm in the face of a difficult situation as opposed to getting upset or depressed.

Jon Kabat-Zinn has clearly had a profound impact on my spiritual growth. His writings have greatly influenced my perspective on change, growth, and my overall well-being. I first came upon his writings in the fall of 1995, a time of great change in my life. *Good Morning America* had just been taken over by the news division of ABC Television after being a part of the entertainment division for twenty years. And ABC Television had just been bought by Disney. The changeover was supposed to be very smooth, and we were told by the news division, "We're not going to change a thing. Trust us." We've all heard those famous words before. All of us, from writers and reporters to directors, producers, and executives, were filled with fear about what changes the new regime would bring not only to the show but to our individual jobs. After all, in one fell swoop we were going to have new bosses. We wondered what the first changes would be.

I was also very well aware that my contract was up for renewal in the upcoming year, which always raises questions of whether "they" (and now I wasn't even sure of who "they" were) will want to renew my contract and whether we will be able to strike a deal. Even without new bosses, that is always a stressful time.

All of us at *GMA* had received a memo requesting us to attend a mandatory reception in the studio immediately after the show one morning. All of the new ABC News executives were going to officially announce the takeover. The hundreds of staff members from the office began to fill the studio. The atmosphere was almost like a party, and yet it didn't feel very festive. Everywhere you went, you heard the same buzz: "Do you think my job's in jeopardy?" "Who do you think is getting fired?" With everyone else worrying, I too began to feel anxious, especially since the newspapers had been speculating for weeks about my future on *GMA,* discussing potential contenders for my spot in the wake of the changeover. While my fears weren't by any means unreasonable, I couldn't help but let them get the best of me that morning.

With a few minutes left before the executives were to arrive, and my fear and uncertainty mounting, I decided to take a necessary time-out. I retreated to my dressing room. As I walked in and shut the door behind me, the first thing I saw was a book I had fortuitously been given the night before, titled *Wherever You Go, There You Are*. It's a book about mindful meditation in everyday life. I opened the book, and by pure chance (or maybe it was meant to be) hit upon a chapter entitled "You Can't Stop the Waves but You Can Learn to Surf." Those words would not only give me a new perspective with which to deal with that day's events but would ultimately change my life forever. The message is that we must all understand that stress is an inevitable part of life. And while we can learn to make intelligent choices to prevent things from becoming worse, there are a lot of things in life over which we have little or no control. But that doesn't mean that we have to be victims. We can learn to work with these new forces, understand them, and use their energies to increase our strength, wisdom, and compassion.

That was the first time that I truly recognized that I could choose how I responded to my set of circumstances. We can be resistant, which only lets stress and fear continue to build. Or we can choose to open ourselves up and be willing to work with whatever it is that lies ahead of us. This kind of acceptance of a situation doesn't mean hanging your head in resignation. It's merely embracing how things are in that moment. And like any wave that inevitably breaks against the shore, you cannot stop it, but you can learn to surf it.

So, with a deep breath, I grabbed my metaphorical board, paddled my way back down to the studio, caught a great big wave, and hung 10! Kowabunga!

As the changeover gradually took place, I began to feel a greater sense of comfort with the new management, and with that came greater self-confidence. I used the changes at work as a motivation to do some very deep work on my own self-awareness, especially regarding the way I respond to change. I have long been a great gatherer of magazine articles. In fact, if you sit next to me on an airplane, be forewarned: I spend most of my time looking for articles that pique my interest and tearing them out one by one. For a long time I would stick those articles in a drawer or make a pile next to my bed. Sure, these

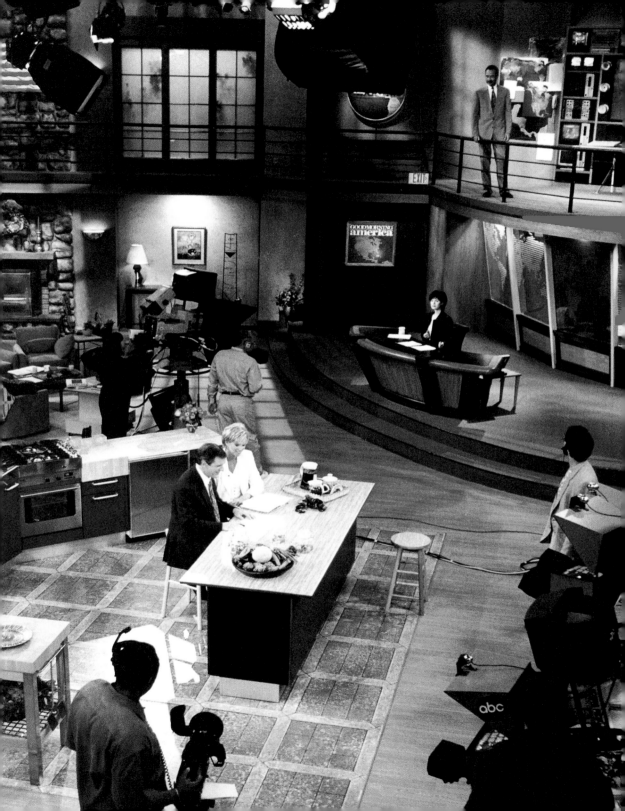

articles all contained jewels of information that I definitely *wanted* to implement into my life, but somehow I never seemed to take the next step and take action with the information. Today, aside from using many of these articles for inspiration and research for this book, I try to *actively incorporate* their wisdom into my life. Reading the information is one thing; using it in your own life is what allows you to grow and become stronger.

As I grew more comfortable at work, I also found I was more confident in speaking my mind. Last year, at a lunch I was attending to get to know some of the new bosses in the news division, I found myself in conversation with one of the top executives. He asked me an interesting question: "What gives one person so much impact on the air and makes another so forgettable?" I smiled as I immediately thought of a magazine article that I had recently read, which contained what I believed to be the perfect answer. But did I dare use it? The article was about the secret to good sex. (All right, get over

Behind the scenes on the set of Good Morning America.

the shock. It's just us girls talking, right?) The author had talked openly with all of her co-workers, her girlfriends, their husbands and boyfriends, and so on. (Funny, they've never given me an assignment like that on *GMA.*) Everyone she talked with had a different response for what constituted the secret. The more people she asked, the more confused the writer became. She wanted to find an expert who would give her the final word on this great mystery of the world, so she finally sought an audience with the Mayflower Madam herself, Sydney Biddle Barrows. When the two women met, Ms. Barrows was able to reveal the secret of good sex (and also her secret of life) in one word: *enthusiasm.*

Needless to say, I was taking a pretty big risk by telling the story. This executive would either love the anecdote or would think that I was absolutely nuts for having this slightly off-color conversation at our first meeting. Luckily I got a great laugh at lunch that day, and maybe even a little respect for my chutzpah! But the point was simple, and I believe he got it: you have to be passionate about whatever it is you do. Bring enthusiasm to everything you take on, and regardless of the results, you will have done the best that you could, and that's all anyone can ask.

The Different Types of Change

Change arrives in many different forms. You can experience change through a crisis: getting divorced, losing your job, changing jobs, or even finding that your kids are all grown up and on their own. Change that occurs through crises is not usually change by choice; it is induced by circumstances or necessity. Most often, this type of change requires a drastic lifestyle modification, resulting in an impact not only on you but on your loved ones as well.

Change can also come out of the drive for self-improvement. This is what I think of as creative intellectual change; it's proactive behavior rather than a response to circumstances. This kind of change usually occurs after you realize that something in your current behavior has become unacceptable to you, and this takes courage. But mostly it is posi-

tive change. It's making a decision to improve your well-being. It can include physical changes that bolster your self-esteem and improve your general health, and internal changes that foster better mental and spiritual health.

Lastly, there are the inevitable changes that come with time, whether we want them or not. The facts are the facts. We all grow older; we all experience changes in our physical appearance and in our mental capacity. I remember reading a great line about this once: "My mind and body are going in the same direction, but not at the same speed." Can you stop the aging process? There are those who think you can. Dr. Deepak Chopra wrote an entire book about it called *Ageless Body, Timeless Mind* in which he contends that changing our expectations and beliefs about growing old can halt and actually reverse the aging process. I'll share his theory in more detail in Chapter 8, in the Golden Years section. One thing's for sure: you can certainly better prepare yourself for these changes that come with age by knowing what to expect and being better prepared to cope with it.

However change is introduced into

your life, you must be willing to try new ideas, accept failure if you don't succeed, and be ready to try a different tack.

Change that occurs through crisis, as its name suggests, is often the most difficult type of change to deal with, as it usually hits your life fast and hard, and it is most often out of your control. My divorce fit into this category. Divorce is never easy, but compound the situation by adding the scrutiny of the media and it becomes overwhelmingly intense. However, a lot of what I've learned comes from enduring those difficult years. Many dramatic and much-needed changes resulted as I dealt with all of the issues of that time of crisis.

There I was, single at forty-one for the first time in seventeen years, only this time I had three kids, a hectic career, and tons of unwanted attention from the press. I felt shy, nervous, and even inadequate as I tried to ready myself for a new life of being on my own, finding a new identity as a single mother, and (gulp) dating. No matter what a woman's age, when she finds herself on her own and reentering the dating scene, she feels like an awkward teenager again, alone and anxious about what comes next.

Most relationship experts I have interviewed on GMA say that it takes from three to five years to get over a divorce or the loss of a spouse. That seemed like forever to me—I just wanted to get on with my life, and I didn't want to believe that it would take that long. In fact, it did take me almost five years. Immediately after the divorce, I threw myself into work and my family (no regrets about that; my children definitely needed my complete attention during this difficult time), and the improved self-esteem I derived from making great strides in my career was much needed at that time. But when I finally put away my work for the day, the kids had gone to sleep, or went off on activities of their own, I could feel something missing in my life. Like many women, I found it easy to come up with excuses not to pursue an active social life. We are very good at convincing ourselves that we don't really need to go out, that we're too busy, that we'd just as soon curl up in front of the television, night after night.

But the truth is, dating after years of being married to one person is just plain scary. So many women I have talked with experienced similar feelings to my own. They worry about how to meet a guy, how to get to know him, how much of themselves to reveal, how to know if he is right for them. They stress about whether or not they are as attractive as they were when they were younger, whether or not they are "desirable," and whether or not they will be able to open themselves up and feel love again. And I was amazed to realize that an issue I had dealt with as a single twenty-something-year-old had resurfaced: being in the public eye, men often assume that I have dates lined up out the door, so they don't think I'll be available, and they don't ask me out. I also had to worry about whether a guy was interested in me for myself, and not because I was a celebrity.

Like many women, I had well-intentioned friends offering to set me up, usually with successful businessmen, which they believed were the proper dates for me. While these men were always nice, and certainly charming and well-mannered, I often felt I was interviewing potential life mates. Why wasn't I just having a night out on the town? I found myself ticking off a guy's attributes, evaluating them for the qualities that I

or (even more insistently) my friends believed they should have. Not exactly a fun, relaxing evening!

Basically I wanted the spontaneity and adrenaline rush of meeting a guy, finding ourselves attracted to each other, and letting things develop naturally, without putting undue pressure on this relationship to "work" or be "going somewhere." Sometimes on a date, by the time the salad had been served, I had already mentally gotten to know the man, progressed through the stages of our relationship, and experienced the disappointment of him not living up to my expectations. And the poor guy was just sipping his wine, without a clue about the mini-drama that had just taken place in my mind!

After months of dating, I finally experienced the impromptu meeting I had been hoping for. When I met Jeff, I understood for the first time what I had been missing in all of those perfect-on-paper dates. Here was a guy who was sweet, unpretentious, considerate, and really seemed to care about me as a person. And his smile! I found myself enjoying the time we were spending together, without feeling the need to

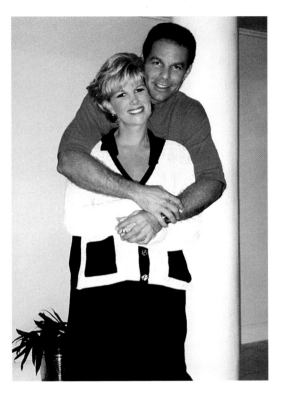

Jeff Konigsberg—he always makes me smile.

assign a definition to the relationship. I could just let it naturally progress. I felt like a woman again, and relearned how to be part of a couple.

I began to realize that I had always allowed myself to be defined by others' perceptions, and that the only person who should be allowed to decide who I am and what I want is me. I began to see more clearly some of my past behaviors,

such as expecting another person to act in exactly the manner I would choose, and my tendency to be quick to assign blame whenever there was a conflict. Now, in this new positive relationship, I was discovering a sort of safe haven in which to examine my actions, and understand my emotions better. Jeff gave me the chance to be me in the context of an adult partnership. Suddenly, dating was a lot more fun than I thought it could ever be! I began to feel less scared, and more excited about trying new things, sharing my feelings, and getting to know this person leisurely.

When you come into a new relationship with preconceived expectations, you are setting yourself up for a fall. You sabotage yourself by not enjoying yourself while you're together because you're too busy judging him; and not allowing either of you the opportunity to get to know each other honestly. Don't trip yourself up! Whether you've been single your whole life, or married before, stop looking for your life partner, and start enjoying yourself. Is getting back out there intimidating? You bet! But when you look at your options, you have to risk a little to gain a lot.

Keep reminding yourself, as I did, "Every date is not a potential husband. Lighten up and have fun!"

> *"The greatest discovery of my generation is that a human being can change his life by changing his attitude of mind."*
> WILLIAM JAMES

If you can identify a problem in your life, you can change the way you react to that problem. Remember, our reaction to a conflict can have a great effect on the outcome.

To create great change and improvement in your life, you must ask for support from others, like family and friends—sometimes a difficult lesson to learn. The more positive energy and reinforcement you have surrounding you, the better the results of your change will be.

Warning: Do realize that sometimes, when you grow as a person, some people around you may have a hard time adapting to these changes, especially when these changes affect them. Sometimes

it's a control issue—for example, your mate may feel that he will no longer have control over you if you lose weight, go back to work, get a degree, and become more independent—or people may feel that you are growing away from them. Sometimes it becomes an issue because your change makes others aware of changes they need to make in their own lives but haven't faced up to yet. Don't let their inertia deter you from staying on your new course. You can ask for their support, but don't assume that your growth will always be easy for everyone else to take.

Let's not forget that we must give support in return, when a friend or loved one is seeking to implement change into her life. Perhaps one of the greatest ways I've been able to give support to other women is through my involvement with the Michael Bolton Foundation. A few years back, Michael asked me to be the mistress of ceremonies for the annual fund-raising dinner and auction for his foundation to benefit abused and battered women. I remembered the support and strength Michael provided to me during my divorce. Through my participation, I knew that I had a chance to

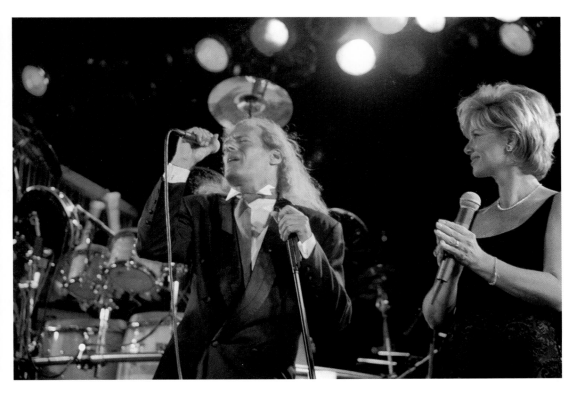

offer, in some small way, the same to
others who needed someone to lean on,
so I gladly accepted his offer to host the
event, and I have done so with great
pride for the last four years.

However, the gift of self-discovery is
one that you must give yourself before

*On stage at the annual Michael Bolton Founda-
tion fund-raiser.*

you can give it to others. And as you
pass along what you've learned, you will
find it reinforces your own journey
toward self-awareness.

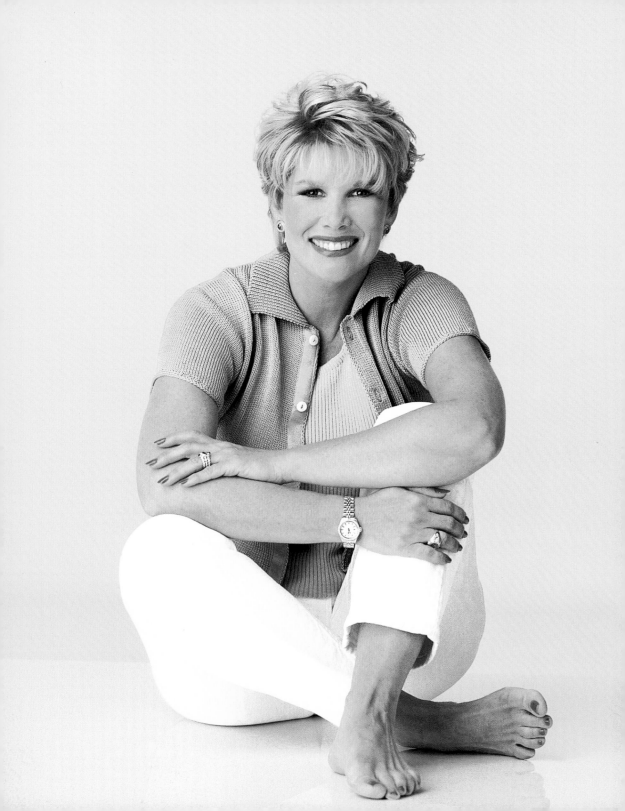

8 Understanding the Cycles of Your Life

Now that we've explored the profound effect that your mind has on your health, we can turn our attention to our physical needs.

Before we address the three essentials of good physical health—nutrition, exercise, and sleep—it's important to have a general understanding of the different cycles of a woman's life. All of us will pass through many stages in our lives and experience many changes in our lifestyles and in our bodies' needs. Recognizing these stages better prepares you to cope with them, and knowing that others experience similar changes offers a much-needed feeling of comfort and community.

"Every age can be enchanting, provided you live within it."

Brigitte Bardot

As our bodies change decade by decade, so do our physical needs and personal challenges. When you're a teenager, you may be able to eat indiscriminately and exercise only every now and then, but developing good nutrition and fitness habits helps lay the foundation for the routines that will be crucial later in life. I only wish that I'd known this when *I* was a teenager!

Today, as a mother of teenage girls, I can help them understand how important it is to manage their health and fitness— for example, that making leaner food choices like more chicken and fish instead of red meat, vegetarian or turkey chili, and of course plenty of fruits and vegetables will put them way ahead of the game

as they get older. And in the meantime, their good eating habits and participation in physical activities will keep them energized and in tip-top shape.

Watching and talking with my daughters and their peers really got me thinking about the traps and challenges we as women face as we move through the stages of our lives.

This chapter will explore these changes and discuss how we can be physically and mentally prepared and continue to be active and vital through all the decades of our lives.

The Teens

I recently asked my sixteen-year-old daughter, Jamie, what health issues were important to her circle of friends. There was one clear theme: fat. They seem to know the fat content of everything we keep in our cupboards. Jamie can tell me the precise number of fat grams in a muffin, a cookie, or a slice of pizza!

She and her friends are all athletic-looking young women. Some of them work out religiously, while some think a dumbbell is what you call your ex-boyfriend. But most of them are thinking more about looking good than getting fit.

So much of how we handle life's challenges and the way we perceive ourselves has its roots in the teen years. Have you noticed how, as girls start to grow into women, they sometimes seem to become less vibrant and curious? They stop playing sports, developing new interests, and making career plans every other day. They start hanging back, affecting an aura of utter boredom, and avoiding conversations about anything more mentally taxing than nail polish.

In her book *Reviving Ophelia: Saving the Selves of Adolescent Girls* Mary Pipher points out that very few girls seem to need psychotherapy from ages seven to eleven. But starting around twelve, girls experience an explosion of unhappiness about themselves and the world around them. Don't think your daughter is immune from feelings of self-doubt and anxiety, even if she doesn't always show them. Though my daughter Jamie is confident and secure most of the time, like most teenagers she also experiences down times. Poetry is her outlet for expressing her deepest thoughts. This is one of the poems she wrote when she was feeling low, and everyone I shared it with was touched by how poignantly she captured her emotions.

It was the most dismal of days
and I was all alone
lonely and sad
just writing a poem

The words flowed out
but all were filled with gloom
I knew I couldn't stay here
so I slowly left my room

There had to be something
to take sadness off my mind
so I reached to the top shelf
to see what I could find

My hand fumbled through
the dust and cobwebs mingled
when suddenly it grabbed something
that sparkled bright and tingled

I pulled it from its spot
upon the shelf high up
and imagine my surprise to find
it was a magic cup!

I took it straight outside
where it was raining, cold, and dim
I stuck my right arm out
and filled my cup to the brim

I watched it for some time
but magic, I saw none
I looked behind a cloud
and saw peeking out, the sun

I looked down at my cup
its ingredients, only one
I decided it needed mixing
from the cup, I let half the liquid run

I raised my head up high
and tightly grasped my cup
floated up to the sun
and brightly filled it up

As I descended back to earth
I watched, amazed to see
a vision of happiness brewing
a rainbow stared back at me!

All the colors sparkled
and my eyes lit up with glee
But with a start I realized
that only my reflection stared back at me.

It was then that I discovered
that only I hold the key
to unlock the true happiness
that lies inside of me

Girls' dissatifaction with themselves also shows up in the way they perform in school. They start to fall behind boys in science and math. Studies found that at the beginning of their teenage years girls and boys scored the same on I.Q. tests. But by the end of the teens, girls' scores had dropped significantly. (It's enough to make you wonder if there's something in the makeup teen girls use.) The focus changes from intellectual achievements to social relationships and physical appearance. These are junk values that can be dangerous: a girl who grows up lacking confidence and feeling insecure is less likely to master the skills she needs to do well in school and prepare for a career. She's also less likely to value her health. We can see this in the rising number of girls who smoke: by eighth grade almost one in five is taking up the habit. Most say they smoke to control their weight. Because of internal anxieties or external pressures, this is the time when physical appearance takes on a greater importance.

WELCOME TO YOUR NEW BODY

Around the age of eleven or twelve, my daughters stopped changing their clothes in front of me and their friends. It's absolutely amazing to watch girls that age maneuver out of one T-shirt and into another so that, God forbid, we (their own mothers!) don't see their boobs. Never mind that we're the ones who fed them, bathed them, and wiped their tushies, for Pete's sake!

As psychologist Dr. Ellen McGrath points out, how a girl reacts to the changes of puberty depends on how her mother handles it. If a mother views the start of menstruation, the budding of breasts, and a rounder shape as symbols of a wonderful step toward adulthood, the daughter will feel a sense of anticipation and excitement about these changes. If Mom shows embarrassment or discomfort, the girl will feel that too—and she'll want to hide the changes of puberty. That can be the start of a very bad body image.

When I took my older daughters to their pediatrician for routine checkups as they entered puberty, I was delighted that the doctor looked them straight in the eye and explained to them that their bodies would be changing a lot over the

next year. Not only would their breasts develop, but their hips would begin to widen. He told them not to view this as getting fat, but rather to see it as developing a more adult shape as they entered womanhood. We as parents must pass this positive attitude along to our daughters, even though they might be embarrassed to hear it.

To help your daughter learn to appreciate her developing body, pay attention to what you say not only about her looks but also your own. What are you teaching her when you moan that you can't fit into your jeans? If you're obsessively talking about wanting to lose weight, your daughter will also be more likely to obsess over her own weight and appearance.

What's the right age for a first visit to the gynecologist? This is sometimes a delicate question for parents of preteen or teenage daughters. During an interview on *GMA,* Dr. Nancy Snyderman said that a good rule of thumb is between the ages of fourteen and sixteen. These girls are experiencing many changes in their bodies, their lives, and the choices confronting them, and they need solid information and reassurance

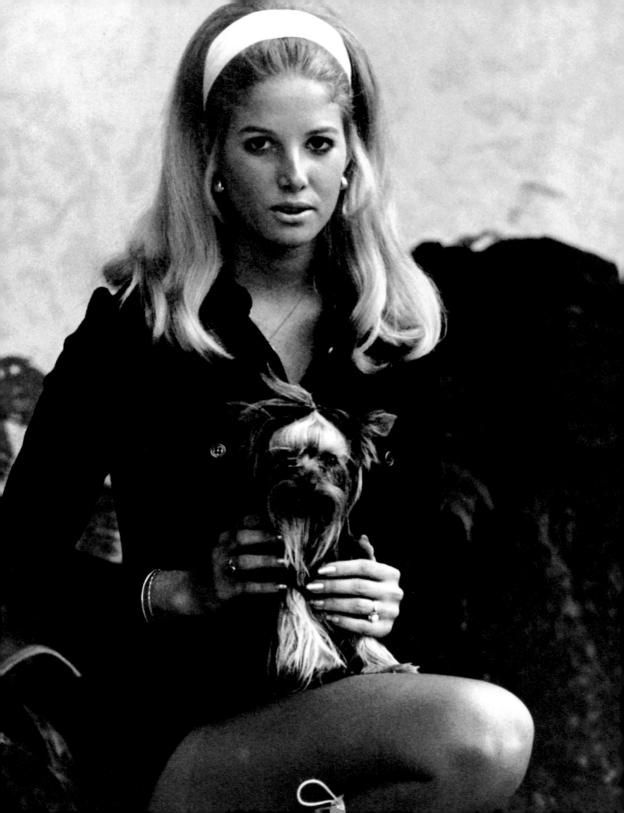

that their bodies are developing just like other girls'. It's important for parents to understand that a visit to the gynecologist does not necessarily mean the start of sexual activity. Young women are interested in understanding their bodies, and this is an excellent opportunity for them to ask questions and get the right answers. Reassure your daughter that her doctor is obligated to keep information confidential so that she can openly share her history and concerns.

Some girls erroneously believe that the changes of puberty prevent them from continuing to be active in sports. It is up to us as parents to show them otherwise. I've encouraged a love for sports in my girls, and all three are very physically active: Jamie is an extremely accomplished competitive equestrian; Lindsay is a dancer (she'd dance ten hours a day if she could); and Sarah, my youngest, is also a dancer, but if she had the time, she would also play hockey, soccer, tennis—and add ice skating and skiing in the winter!

Besides giving them a sense of sportsmanship and self-confidence, sports are a wonderful way to exercise. Being over-

Me at sixteen.

weight is tough for an adult and much more so for a vulnerable kid trying to navigate her way through adolescence. Childhood obesity is definitely on the rise (about 25 percent of our kids are now officially fat), largely because kids spend too much time lounging on the sofa.

THE MENSTRUAL CYCLE

The start of menstruation can be embarrassing and scary, even for girls who seem to be blasé. The average American girl has her first period around age thirteen, but it can be several years earlier or later. If she starts menstruating before age nine or hasn't started by age sixteen, she should see a doctor, just to be sure all is well.

If a girl feels anxious because many of her friends have gotten their period, a doctor can reassure her that she is normal, and although there is probably nothing to worry about, a doctor's reassurance may make her feel better.

The length and heaviness of each woman's menstruation is different, and can vary from month to month, and she may have concerns about her own menstrual cycle as well.

According to Nancy Snyderman, the medical correspondent for *GMA* and

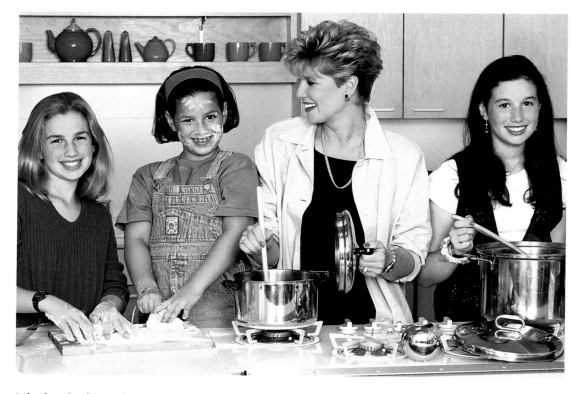

The family that cooks together, makes a mess together! If you think this is bad, you ought to see my teenagers' rooms.

author of *Dr. Nancy Snyderman's Guide to Good Health,* most menstruating women will suffer some form of PMS. There has been a great deal of controversy about what PMS is and what causes it. We've talked often about it on *GMA* and posed questions to Dr. Snyderman, who has a way of presenting material that helps

put it in perspective and clarifies the information.

For instance, she says that the term "raging hormones" has "dogged the path of women's emancipation for decades," and it's time to lay this phrase to rest once and for all.

"Hormones do not rage," says Dr. Snyderman. "Hormone levels in the body change as they are designed to... it's natural and it's our biology." She says the most common physical symptoms of

PMS are breast tenderness, a craving for salt or sweets, abdominal bloating, headaches, and leg swelling. You may also notice fatigue, nausea, diarrhea, or constipation. The most common psychological symptoms, according to Dr. Snyderman, include irritability, a sense of things not quite working right or going right or being right, depression, a loss of self-confidence, and hostility. Basically, PMS is a somewhat predictable pattern of changes, physical and emotional, that some women experience just before their monthly period. These symptoms vary from woman to woman and from month to month.

For women who suffer these symptoms on a regular basis, Nancy suggests keeping a chart for a couple of months. The chart should track the number of days you menstruate and the heaviness of your flow. Record your thoughts, moods, headaches, and food cravings or intolerances. She then recommends you share this information with your doctor, who might prescribe medications to alleviate the symptoms: diuretics to alleviate bloating; Progesterone to be taken orally or vaginally; or even an antidepressant such as Xanax or Prozac.

More recently it's been discovered that PMS might also be due in part to a deficiency of the naturally produced chemical serotonin. So it makes sense that certain medications (like Prozac) that inhibit the uptake of serotonin by the body would help alleviate PMS symptoms.

Dr. Snyderman has always urged women not to underestimate the effect of a good diet and exercise during menstruation. Many women find that adding a morning exercise routine in particular helps relieve some of the tension and symptoms of PMS. Others find that taking acetaminophen, such as Tylenol, or ibuprophen, such as Advil, for a few nights before their period is due helps relieve discomfort.

With her usual commonsense approach, Dr. Snyderman has always urged our female viewers to try behavior changes before seeking a solution through medications.

PMS RELIEF DIET TIPS

Whether you have a little PMS or a lot, changing what you eat could help you feel better. Dr. Snyderman suggests the following tips to counteract the symptoms of PMS:

1. Halt the salt! Eating foods containing a lot of salt in the days before your period can cause bloating. Stay away from canned soups, processed foods, and salted snacks.

2. Eliminate caffeine. Going easy on caffeine may reduce irritability. This includes coffee, tea, and colas that contain caffeine.

3 Eliminate refined sugar and refined flour products.

4. Reduce or eliminate alcohol.

5. Increase your water intake.

6. Eat more protein and fewer carbohydrates. Large amounts of protein-rich food induce fluid loss, which reduces bloating; in contrast, carbs are stored in the body and cause you to retain water. Try to stick with complex carbohydrates such as whole grain foods and fresh produce, which are easier to process than simple carbohydrates.

7. Avoid carbonated drinks. They introduce air into your body through those tiny bubbles and can cause bloating and gas. Even bubbly water can do this, so be careful.

8. Avoid constipating foods such as rice, mashed potatoes, pasta, and boiled chicken. Instead, munch on small amounts of fiber-filled fruits, like apples, pears, and prunes.

9. Watch your fat intake.

10. Stay away from chocolate. Not only is it high in fat and calories but it can also cause mood swings as well.

11. Look for foods rich in B_6 vitamins. Eat lean meats, chicken, fish, rice, and beans, which keep your energy level up. Also include in your diet foods with iron, zinc, and magnesium, like liver, poultry, eggs, tomatoes, broccoli, lettuce, mushrooms, and onions.

TEENS AND SEXUALITY

Passing through puberty also means the first awareness of sexuality and the possibility of sexual exploration. This brings with it the risk of sexually transmitted diseases (STDs) and early pregnancy. Surveys done in the 1940s found that only about 10 percent of girls had had intercourse by age sixteen; surveys done in the 1990s found that *half* of the girls had had sex. Most of us hope that our daughters will postpone sex until they're older, but at any age unprotected sex is a serious health risk. It's not hypocritical to tell your daughter, "I don't want you to have sex; I don't think you're ready. Your safety and health are my biggest concerns." Then make sure she knows how to protect herself from pregnancy and STDs, especially HIV. If you are uncomfortable discussing sex with your daughter, set up an appointment for her with your family doctor or gynecologist so that she will receive accurate information and feel free to ask questions. And keep reminding yourself that despite the pierced noses and purple hair, most teenagers hold the same values as their parents.

To help your daughter build a strong foundation for a life of physical and emotional well-being, remember that knowledge is power. Books such as Dr. Pipher's *Reviving Ophelia* and *All That She Can Be* by Dr. Carol Eagle and Carol Colman can be helpful in teaching you how to encourage your daughter to grow. For you former hippies, I recommend *Getting Your Kids to Say "No" in the Nineties When You Said "Yes" in the Sixties* by Dr. Victor Strasburger.

Leaving the Nest

When young people move out of their parents' home, whether to go off to college or get a new apartment, they face a whole new set of challenges. A lot of young adults are not prepared for this new independence: getting themselves up and out in the morning, organizing their time, budgeting their money, getting enough sleep at night, and so on.

Colleges don't take on a substitute-parent role anymore; the students are expected to be responsible for themselves. Young adults are faced with a lot of new temptations, without parents around to intercede. Students, particularly freshmen, may have a difficult time with new responsibilities such as handling credit cards and prioritizing their schedules. The only way to try to prevent problems is to discuss potential pitfalls with them before they leave.

College triggers major anxiety in many young women. Part of the problem may be girls' tendency to attribute their success to luck, while boys more often credit their skills. "We see what's called the impostor phenomenon," says Dr. McGrath. "They're not sure they're smart enough; or maybe they don't really belong there. Some girls actually wonder if they were admitted by mistake!"

GETTING INTO THE CHECKUP HABIT

Young adulthood is a good time to start the habit of routine medical checkups. Here are the basics:

- *Find a doctor you trust. If you don't feel comfortable, you might not want to talk about that "personal" rash or lump, and that could be dangerous. No one should die of embarrassment.*

- *Get an annual breast exam and ask your doctor to teach you how to do breast self-exam. Do it each month the week after your period.*

- *If you have ever had unprotected sex (without a condom), ask to be tested for STDs (sexually transmitted diseases), including an HIV, or AIDS, test. You could have one of these without knowing it. Untreated chlamydia or gonorrhea could leave you sterile, and AIDS is much more serious.*

- *Ask for copies of any lab test results. That lets you double-check for mistakes, such as a mix-up of your test with someone else's, and helps you keep track of your tests and results. If anything is unusual, make a follow-up appointment right away and ask the doctor if she has any printed information about the problem.*

- *Ask questions! Am I getting enough calcium? Do I need a Pap smear or any other tests? Are there new birth control options I should know about? Bring a list of questions with you and take notes during the appointment. It's even okay to ask what things will cost or to ask for another opinion. This is not a social situation. And who else will watch out for your health if you don't?*

THE FRESHMAN 15

The first year or two of college is a high-risk time for a woman's weight as well as for her self-image. All those snack-fueled late-nighters contribute to what is called the "freshman 15." The specific cause of this weight gain, according to experts such as Dr. McGrath, is a combination of opportunity and anxiety.

College is the first time young women are totally on their own in making food choices. "Now, at two o'clock in the morning, you can go out with friends for pizza," says dietitian Michelle Daum, author of *A Can Do Eating Plan for Overweight Kids and Teens.* "Right down the hall is a vending machine. You may be up until three o'clock in the morning and sleep until noon every day. So your schedule is changed, you may be eating more sporadically, and you're confronted with opportunities to eat that weren't there before." It's fine to go out for pizza with friends, as long as it's not every night. Renting a mini-fridge and stocking it with fruit and nonfat yogurt for study snacks and quickie breakfasts is a smart idea nutritionally and economically. Skipping meals is a setup for pigging out on junk later.

The combination of studying and socializing and the pressures they induce often lead to less sleep. "For a lot of people, the signals are crossed between fatigue and hunger," says Dr. James Rippe, associate professor at Tufts University School of Medicine. This increases the temptation of late-night snacking. Throw in homesickness, boredom, television watching, a lot of food commercials, and it's easy to see how nonstop munching becomes a threat. "Bulimia becomes another extracurricular activity in some sororities," reports Dr. Ellen McGrath. "It becomes a way to indulge but also manage weight. Anorexia (self-starvation) and bulimia (bingeing and purging) are very serious stuff and can lead to everything from digestive and kidney problems to damaged teeth and bones to heart failure."

Having more alcohol around raises the risks for young women. Binge drinking is rampant on college campuses. In a survey of college students in Massachusetts, one-third of the girls reported that at some point in the last two weeks they'd downed five or more drinks in a row! "In our laboratory, when we have people do food diaries, we treat alcohol basically as a fat," says Dr. Rippe, a cardiologist. "In terms of how your body handles the calories, think of that glass of wine as though you're drinking a glass of olive oil." Yecch! And of course drinking a lot of alcohol isn't just a threat to the waistline; it can also become a serious health issue, and can cause big problems in your work and your life.

It's important to know the risks of poor and dangerous habits and to plan coping strategies ahead of time. Often young women begin what can become chronic lifelong habits, or even addictions, by turning to food and alcohol to try to suppress feelings of anxiety, loneliness, or depression. Once the habits become a learned mechanism, they are harder to stop, and they become even more difficult to control later in life. Management techniques, like the ones in Chapter 5, are useful in combatting anxieties in a healthy, healing manner.

Building new social support is another must for a freshman's emotional health. A group of watchful friends who share her values can feel like a second family. Staying connected to home through telephone calls, letters, e-mail, and "care packages" will also ease that sense of isolation. It's especially important for you as a parent to allow your daughter to vent her fears and frustrations. Encourage her to use campus resources for help (most colleges have counselors and even support groups available), and remind her that you're always there for her, even if you think she already knows it.

Juggling It All

Life is tougher than ever for young women today. The job market is so complex and changes so fast that the training a student gets today could well be obsolete in the job market tomorrow, before that tuition loan is paid off. A woman on her own for the first time has to be flexible and anticipate constant flux.

I can certainly speak to this one! Being the new kid on the block when I first came to New York as a cub reporter for WABC-TV, I was usually called in first at 6:00 A.M. and let out last after the 11:00 P.M. news. Oh, sure, I was making a nice salary working in the Big Apple,

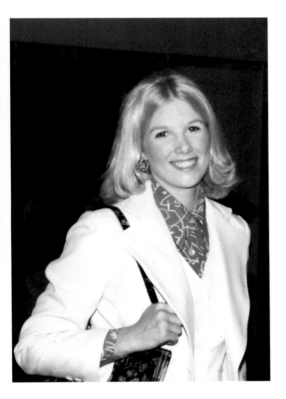

On assignment during my first few days of work in New York City.

but when was I supposed to spend it? I had no time to shop, dine out, or go to the theater—all of those wonderful things I had heard about New York City life. Most nights it was me, my pullout sofa, my cat, and a TV dinner.... So much for the glamorous world of New York television!

The first step in managing this new independence is understanding that it's going to be difficult. You're striving to master the skills you need for your job, and you're probably gaining self-esteem from your work. You're learning to run your new home—or, more likely, your small apartment. You're cooking, cleaning, grocery shopping...and did I forget to mention building a social life? In other words, young women have to learn several sets of skills at once and then try to integrate them.

By the end of their twenties, most women will have mastered some of these basic life skills and will have chosen a direction in terms of career and relationships. "You put the identity blocks together in the twenties," says Dr. Ellen McGrath. "The thirties are when you feel the identities clash with each other, and hopefully learn to make some kind of peace with both sides."

Love and Marriage

When a woman gets married, she makes an active commitment to share a life, to form a partnership with another person. This may be the moment when she

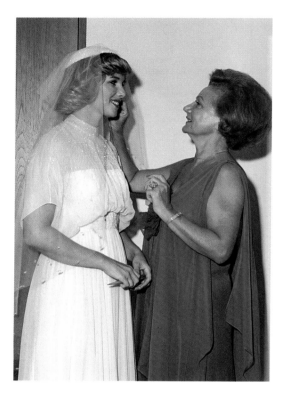

My mom and me on my wedding day.

That's right, even the most driven working girl may soon find herself automatically taking responsibility for everything from cleaning the toilet to cooking. She may somehow feel she has to take care of other people, especially her spouse, since she has taken on this new adult role. I think a good reminder of what role women have *not* taken on can be found in the lyrics of Alanis Morissette's "Not the Doctor": "I don't want to be your mother—I didn't carry you in my womb for nine months."

Both partners had better sit down and talk openly about what they expect from each other and from themselves in their new roles. They might negotiate for their least-hated chores: he cooks most dinners, and she handles all the laundry. These are good preventative tactics.

Researchers say that the way couples disagree (okay—fight) has a lot to do with whether a marriage will last. If there is a problem, set a time and place to talk it out. Explain the details of the problem: when it occurred and how each person felt. Each spouse should ask the other to restate his or her point of view to ensure an understanding of each other's feelings. Then the couple

finally feels that she has grown up and found her adult home: physically, socially, and emotionally. Hold on to that word "partnership," because a marriage has to be a cooperative, give-and-take effort. Unfortunately, even for women who spent their twenties searching for independence, it can be surprisingly easy to slip into the traditional female role of helpmate and supporting cast.

should brainstorm solutions together and try to schedule another time to review whether the plan worked. John Gottman, a psychologist at the University of Washington, offers this rule of thumb: if a couple has about five loving or kind exchanges for every blowup, complaint, or put-down, they'll do okay together.

THE NEWLYWED SPREAD

With marriage, I found myself in the kitchen on a more regular basis. And making nice home-cooked meals for my husband meant constant tasting and sampling, of course. I became practically a hostage of my cupboards and refrigerator. At any given moment it was a challenge not to succumb to their temptations. As I cooked, I would consume an entire meal before I ever sat down at the table! I never seemed to include those taste tests when counting up my daily caloric intake, but they do count, and they definitely add up, down, and all around, and I do mean round.

It's not just sliding into bad habits that adds pounds as you get older. Most people lose muscle mass with age, and muscle burns more calories than fat. Without regular strength training to maintain muscles, the metabolism will slow by roughly 5 percent each decade.

"Your body requires fewer and fewer calories every year past about your mid-twenties," dietitian Michelle Daum says. "The effect of it starts to become noticeable for women probably somewhere in their thirties. They suddenly have this awakening where they say, 'Gee, I'm not eating any differently than before, but I'm sure gaining weight!'

"Well, the reason is you don't need as much food as you did before. You don't need at thirty-five what you needed at twenty-five. This is the hardest advice for people to accept."

So that women and their spouses don't view exercise as something that takes time away from their marriage, it's nice to find one or two sports—even walking or biking—that both people enjoy. This can also strengthen a marriage; for men, doing stuff together (not just talking) is the key to closeness. But women must schedule regular exercise into their lives—even if their mates do not. Women must make their own health a priority.

Pregnancy and Motherhood

When babies enter the picture, oh, baby, baby, fasten your seat belt (really loose), 'cause it's gonna be a bumpy ride! A woman's body goes through an amazing metamorphosis. It's not just the expansion of the tummy. The hips spread, too, and the tush takes on a whole new dimension, practically needing its own zip code. And if women gain enough weight, their feet get larger and their hands swell. My shoe size increased with each pregnancy!

During pregnancy, the body goes through a whole series of hormonal changes, which may cause fluid retention and food cravings. That's nature's way of getting you to do all the things necessary to nourish your baby correctly. Women have to accept the fact that their bodies are changing for a reason and that the goal is to keep the mother and the baby healthy.

"I often see people really having terrible eating disorders when they're pregnant," says fitness expert Barbara Brandt, "because they have worked so hard to achieve a certain body, and they're unwilling to let it go. They don't look at the larger picture of what it's

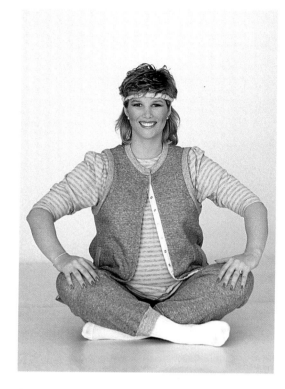

doing to their child, because they can't get past a negative body image."

Doctors stress that it's both healthy and important to gain some weight during pregnancy. "You need to pay attention to what your doctor says about how much weight to gain when you're pregnant," says Dr. James Rippe. More important, women need to make sure they're eating healthy foods. They should ask their doctor about vitamin supplements. And pregnancy shouldn't

OH, NO—STRETCH MARKS!

As if all the other stresses that go with motherhood aren't enough, Mother Nature bestows the gift of pinkish or reddish brown streaks on the bellies and breasts of at least half of pregnant women. Some of us even get them around the thighs, rear, upper arms, and groin.

These (expletive deleted) stretch marks happen when fast growth stretches your skin too far, tearing the collagen and elastin fibers. The tendency to get them runs in families, and all the vitamins, lotions, and special support garments in the world don't seem to prevent them.

The question is, can you get rid of them? We asked that question of Dr. Nancy Snyderman on *Good Morning America.* Her answer: "Not completely, but partially." Stretch marks will fade to pale silver over time. A doctor can prescribe Retin-A cream, which may shrink them somewhat. The newest treatment is laser resurfacing, which removes the topmost layer of your skin. If you want to try this, be sure to go to a very experienced doctor.

be used as an excuse to form high-fat snacking habits that might be hard to change after the baby's delivered.

Most of us, when we think of pregnancy, focus on the physical changes—a swelling belly, tender breasts, and bouts of morning sickness—and pay less attention to the emotional changes. But what's going on inside our heads during pregnancy is at least as important.

Many women find they are much more emotional and more forgetful than they were before they got pregnant. You shouldn't be surprised if you suddenly start crying at sappy movies or when you hear certain song lyrics, or flare into anger over little things and then feel overwhelmed by remorse. No, you're not going crazy! It's just that your body is flooded with all sorts of hormones that affect, among other things, how intensely you feel. To help with forgetfulness, carry around a small notebook—and try not to forget where you put it!

Psychologist Lawrence Kutner, author of *Pregnancy and Your Baby's First Year,* shared with me this excellent advice on how to make it through the tough parts: "One of the best gifts a pregnant couple can give each other is increased tolerance and forgiveness." Pregnancy is also a time for planning. I'm not just talking about how to decorate the baby's room or worrying about paying for his or her college education. You will have some important decisions to make as a couple. Dr. Kutner reiterates the five issues a pregnant couple should discuss early on:

◆ What things will you let slide at home during and after the pregnancy? Most first-time parents underestimate how totally and overwhelmingly exhausted they'll be at the end of pregnancy and during the baby's first year. Forget about keeping the house immaculate and cooking gourmet dinners for a while. Learn to ignore the dust and order a bit more take-out than you used to.

◆ How much time will each of you take off from work before and after your baby is born? You shouldn't be the only one staying home at the beginning!

◆ If both of you will be returning to work, how will you do that? Will one of you take a part-time job—at least at first? Will you share a job with someone else? Will you both work the same shift?

◆ Look into child care if one of you won't be staying at home full-time. No, it's not too early! In fact, one of the toughest challenges the parents of newborns face is finding good (and safe!) child care. Don't wait to start shopping around.

◆ Talk about any religious training or ceremonies you would like your child to have. If you have a boy, will he be circumcised, and by whom? Should your baby have a formal christening? Discuss this even if you and your spouse come from the same religious background. You'll be surprised how often parents carry around different assumptions about religion and ceremonies. If you haven't already discussed these issues, it is important to do so now.

THOSE FIRST MONTHS WITH A BABY

After those nine long months of pregnancy, there is that incomparable moment when a new mother first holds her baby. Finally meeting a newborn baby face-to-face—seeing and touching all her tiny, exquisite parts—is a real rush. It never seems like anything less than a miracle.

I think that most first-time mothers, including me, fear that they might drop her, break her, forget her, underfeed her, overfeed her....One minute you're just a couple, and the next (okay, maybe it's more like fifteen hours later), you're a family!

If ever there is a time when a woman needs support and a boost of self-esteem, it's right after pregnancy. She is always so busy caring for the new baby and seeing to the needs of her other children, she needs a little time for herself and her spouse.

Unfortunately, the rush of hormones that accompanies the process of giving birth can leave a woman feeling lousy. "About 60 to 80 percent of the time after a woman has had a baby, she will have a huge emotional letdown," says Dr. Ellen McGrath. This is called postpartum depression.

Women often feel despair, but this is a very normal, albeit unpleasant and sometimes scary, experience. A typical thought might be "I don't see how I'll ever lose this weight" or "I can't remember what it felt like to have energy." They might even worry that they're losing it: "I can't handle this! I'm falling apart!" Although this period of depression will vary in length, women usually feel significantly better within a couple of weeks. If not, they should talk to a doctor to see if they need treatment.

Even if a woman feels pretty good after the birth, caring for a new baby is very demanding. Those first few months mean constant activity and not nearly enough sleep. A lot of crying—by the

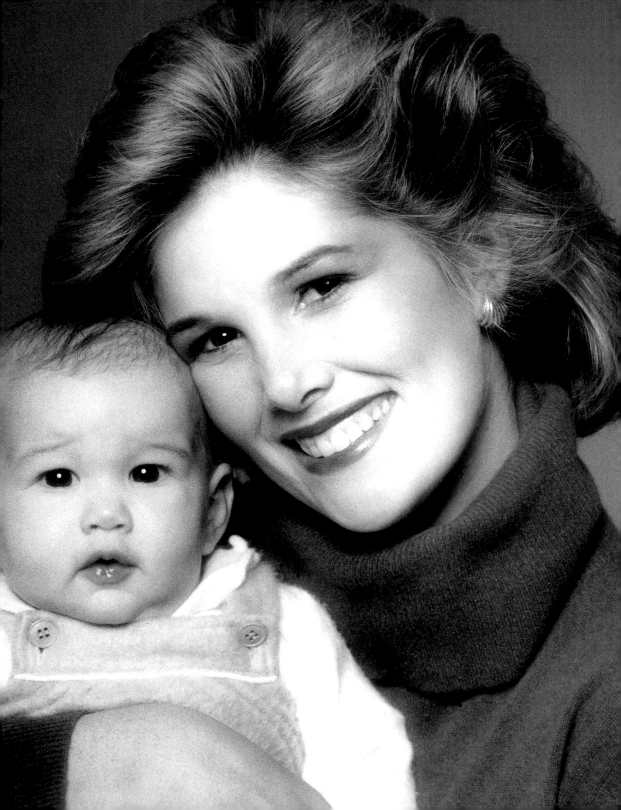

baby, but also some by the mother!—is normal. By about the third month, when those coos and smiles start, it becomes easier to remember why they wanted to be mothers.

After the baby is born, for many women it can be shock to see how much extra flab they're still wearing. This is no time for complacency. "We have this societal expectation that some of that weight that you gain will remain on," explains Dr. Rippe, author of *Fit Over Forty.* "But there is no reason, if you get physically active and pay attention to good eating principles, why you should not be able to get back to your pre-pregnancy weight."

What's more, says Dr. Rippe, "There's very good data from the Nurses Cooperative Trial, a twenty-year ongoing study of 110,000 women, that it is hazardous to your health, in terms of increasing your risk of both cardiovascular disease and cancer, if you gain weight during pregnancy and don't take it off afterward.

"Within a few months after pregnancy, you reestablish your menstrual periods, and all those hormonal changes

Little Jamie in 1980. The true meaning of joy . . . getting to know your new baby.

stabilize," Dr. Rippe continues. "And the reason that people don't lose the weight is the stress of the new baby, the disruption in daily patterns, and all the eating cues. It really is a cultural thing rather than a metabolic thing."

For a lot of women, says dietitian Michelle Daum, "their ideal weight is what they were when they were married. That's the magic number people hold in their heads." She believes that unrealistic goals set women up for frustration, yo-yo dieting, and failure. And they shouldn't fall into the trap of crash dieting. "It took a long time for you to get to this point," Daum says. "And you're not gonna lose it in three weeks!"

While being handed a new baby is a scary proposition, women also realize they are being handed a wonderful opportunity to develop parts of themselves that they never dreamed were there. They learn about the joy of looking at things in a fresh way, through the eyes of a child. But they also have to be realistic about the stress of becoming a parent as their role overload—and usually their role conflict as well—is greatly increased.

Two-thirds of American moms are now in the paid labor force. Psychologists find that no matter what combination of career and homemaking women choose, they never feel that they've found the right balance. They must try to accept that they will never feel as if they've got it all. If they work and rely on a caregiver, they feel guilty that they're not at home. If they're home, at times they'll feel as if they're left out of what's really happening.

The Big Four-Oh!

> *"Nothing great happens until after you're forty."*
> COCO CHANEL

As women approach their forties, they often find themselves exploring, clarifying, and "owning" their values. Most of them have made up their minds about what they find important in life. They feel much more secure, confident, and interested in trying some new things. It's a harvesting age, when they start to reap the benefits of all the hard work and

soul-searching they did earlier in their lives, and now they're able to enjoy themselves more.

Many of us enter this phase of our lives around the time that our children start their teenage years, which brings its own set of challenges. When psychologist Laurence Steinberg interviewed mothers for his book *Crossing Paths,* he expected to hear them talk about how sad they were to think of their children getting ready to leave the nest. Surprisingly, most told him how excited they were as they prepared for that time of new freedom. "If anything, it was living with an adolescent child, not anticipating the child's departure, that was the cause of distress," Dr. Steinberg wrote. (Not that *I've* ever felt that way!)

However, it's somewhat ironic that while they may be experiencing a new sense of freedom, women do feel a tinge of sadnes as well because their kids may not seem to need them in the same way. But this is a time to remodel their lives and reinvent themselves. While this is exciting, it also can be scary. As certain things change in their lives, they can

On top of the world!

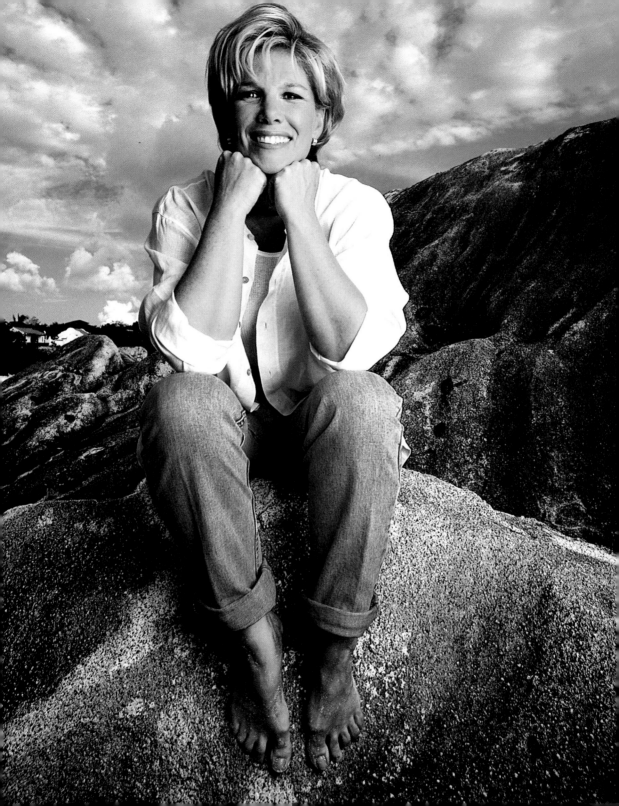

choose to leave those spaces empty or fill them with new people and activities that stimulate them and bring them pleasure. This transition will be easier if they have prepared for it by taking care of their physical health and maintaining relationships outside of their family. If I had to choose one word to sum up this decade, it would be "assessment." This is a time of evaluation, reflection, and change.

Elizabeth Dole, a true trailblazer for women in government, is a good example of a woman who, in her forties, felt that her life had become unbalanced. She realized that her career had taken over her life, and she had what she describes as a spiritual awakening: "I wanted to shift those priorities so that my faith would be at the center again." During speeches Dole tells her audiences that God had gotten lost in her Rolodex somewhere between gardening and government. She goes on to say that "if you're not marching to your own tune, you're going to be marching to someone else's. You have to take control of your own life, set your own priorities, or someone will be happy to set them for you."

Many women in their forties feel as if this is a time to take a new kind of responsibility for themselves to grow up in a different way. And there's another dose of reality that often hits at this time: economic reality. Women in their forties have usually worked fewer hours than their male counterparts and have less "value" in the marketplace. And on the whole women outlive men and therefore have more years to prepare for. The main point? Don't wait. Even women who are now financially solvent must face up to the hard fact that one out of two women get divorced and that most of the ones who remain married will outlive their husbands. Sadly, many women have not been the ones handling the household's finances, and must educate themselves about economics, the sooner the better. Often women wait for a crisis to hit to learn what's what with their finances. In fact, they should be aware of their financial situation from the start, to avoid a monetary crisis and just because it is *their* future, and therefore the responsibility is theirs. Another big issue women in particular tend to avoid is the creation of a will. Again, this is something they need to do to make sure

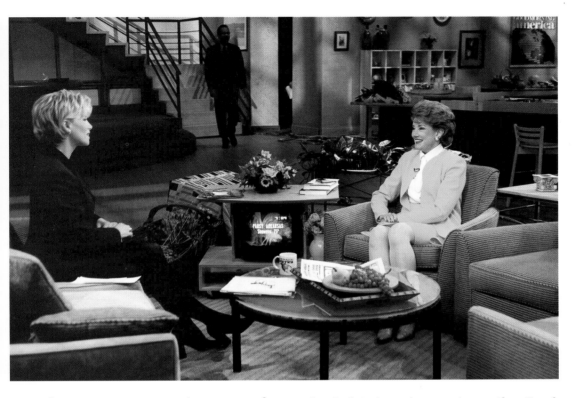

Elizabeth Dole on the campaign trail at Good Morning America.

their best interests are taken care of, and only each individual woman can know what those are.

While women shouldn't wait until their forties to deal with these issues, this is the time when many women first find the time to learn about and take control of their finances. Unsure of how to begin? Head for your local bookstore and check out the shelves of books and workbooks that will help you get started.

CELEBRATING A NEW BEGINNING

With the importance our society places on youth for its own sake, it is sometimes difficult to appreciate the richness of experience that a woman in her forties possesses. We must not allow ourselves to be devalued just because our butts aren't as tight as a twenty-something-

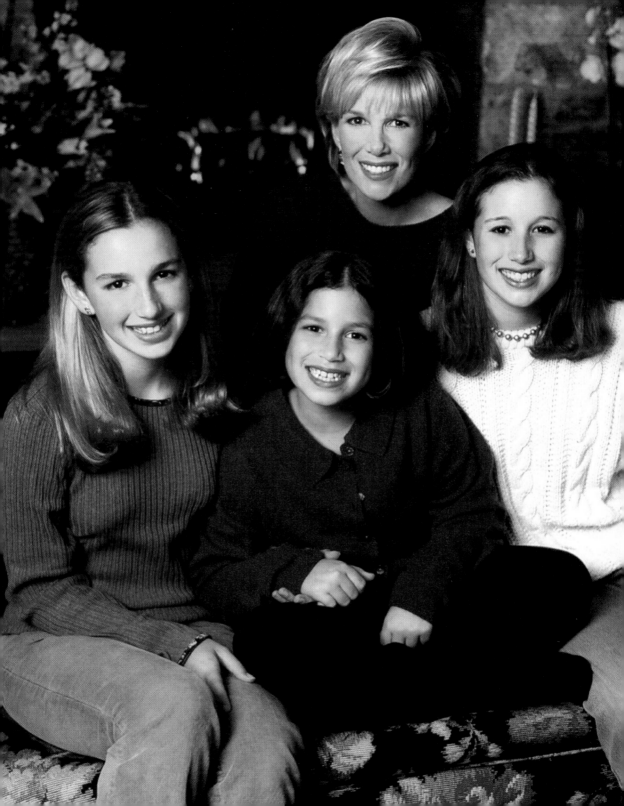

year-old's. I entered my forties taking better care of my body than ever before. I finally figured out that the object was not to look like a twenty-five-year-old, but to look like a healthy, energetic, life-loving woman. Women should celebrate the things they know that they didn't know before, the goals they have achieved, and the circle of family and friends that they have created.

Life Begins at Fifty

"One of the many things nobody ever tells you about middle age is that it's such a nice change from being young."

DOROTHY CANFIELD FISHER

Another life really does begin at fifty. With the incredible advances in science and medicine in the last seventy-five years, our average life expectancy has increased from fifty-four to seventy-six years, and it continues to expand. Of course, that challenges us as individuals

In my forties, life with my girls is better than ever.

to make those extra years the healthiest and happiest they can be. New possibilities open before women. This is the age when they gain the freedom and confidence to pursue their passions, the things that give their lives real meaning —not to mention fun. If there is one concept that epitomizes what women have to do to be healthy, it would be "activity." Not just physical activity but finding ways to keep their minds active as well. Women should ask themselves what they have always wanted to do: maybe it's teaching adults to read or advocating childrens' rights. It's a good time to reintroduce childhood hobbies or sports into their lives as well.

In *In Style* magazine, June 1996, Goldie Hawn had this to say about turning fifty:

I'm making the most of everything. I feel better than ever. I feel more sexually charged than ever. I feel more inspired than ever. And the good news is, I know who I am and I'm very proud of what I've accomplished. Now my focus is moving on to the next stage of my life. And that is about who I want to be at sixty, who I want to be at seventy, who I want to be at eighty. I want to move in a fashion that helps me through the transition

MENOPAUSE

Menopause can arrive as early as forty or as late as sixty. Most women start noticing the onset of the physical and emotional changes of menopause toward fifty: irritability, forgetfulness, mood swings, insomnia, and hot flashes due to a reduction of estrogen in the body. While "menopause" means that menstrual periods stop, it's not a quick and simple process. Like puberty, when all this hormone action started, the winding down of fertility happens over a period of years, and both transitions feature hormone-induced symptoms.

"I think the biggest issue that women face during menopause is the feeling of loss of control over their body," says Dr. James Rippe, author of *Fit Over Forty*. "One way that you can combat that is to do things that say, 'I am, to a large degree, in control of my body.' Regular exercise is one of the very best things you can do to combat this sense that your body's out of control."

of letting go of motherhood and moving into my womanhood. Using my feminine power, my feminine energy, to continue to express myself. To teach and learn and accomplish things. I still have a lot to do.

With the children "launched" and a clearer set of values, this a woman's opportunity to take on the world. Pursuing passions is also a way to cope with the losses that go hand in hand with aging. There are the physical losses: women may not be able to do as much as

they used to do, and they're more vulnerable to conditions like heart disease and osteoporosis. There are also emotional losses. This is often the time when people lose their parents, or even a friend. And since women live longer than men and tend to marry someone older, most of them will spend some years as widows. But the fuller a woman's life is, and the more passions and interests she is actively pursuing, the less these losses will impede her ability to enjoy life.

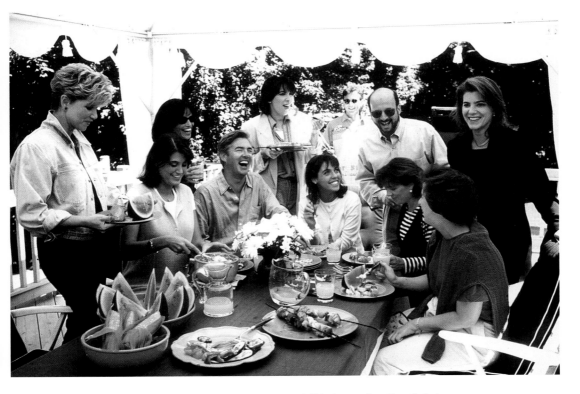

Creating a Family of Choice

By this stage of life, many women have also assembled a family of choice—that is, a group of people they love and care about as if they were family members. Women devote time to developing and maintaining these relationships, and the members of the group support each other at times of vulnerability. This family helps them keep it all together and really makes their lives worth living.

This is my family of choice.

> **"It's the friends you can call at 4:00 a.m. that matter."**
> MARLENE DIETRICH

I certainly know the immeasurable benefits of creating a family of choice. With an extremely small extended family, all of whom live far away, I have a circle of close friends who fill the roles of family members. And for my children, they are essentially aunts and uncles. (In some cases, kids swear they have two or three mothers and a couple of dads as well!) I consider us all very lucky to have this close and loving family of choice.

The Golden Years

"Old age ain't for sissies."
BETTE DAVIS

We are fortunate to live in a time when women are redefining themselves, taking on new roles and challenges, and enjoying longer lives to fit it all in. We need to make each decade count. Women mustn't get stuck in a rut and think, "Wasn't it great when I was a kid (or when I was in college or before I had children) and had time to enjoy life?" What's so different about today? We can all relearn how to enjoy it.

People don't grow old. When they stop growing, they become old.

When I first read these words written by Deepak Chopra in his best-selling book *Ageless Body, Timeless Mind*, I thought to myself, "What an optimist." Still, I couldn't resist buying a copy. Deepak Chopra challenges our long held concept of being old and defies us to ever think of aging the same way again. I was reminded of his words recently upon hearing a friend who's in her late seventies say, "Whoever called these the 'golden years' was full of baloney. I just don't have my pep and pizzazz anymore. I ache all over. I feel like my get-up-and-go has got up and gone. I'm tired, I'm depressed, and I'm lonely." Another friend was recently talking about her grandparents. Her grandfather, trying to make his wife's life easier, hired a driver for her and a full-time live-in housekeeper. My friend's grandmother was not invalid, nor was she incapable of doing these things for herself. Although her husband's intentions were good, the reduction in her independence became debilitating. She was left with nothing to do but grow old. My friend said that in the six months her grandmother has had the extra help, she has aged a decade.

It's frightening to watch older people

give up their desire for life. In his book, Deepak Chopra warns that "when life becomes meaningless the body's sustaining energy seems to drain silently away, like a leaky battery. But if we look closer, we can prove that this draining away of vitality, curiosity, and the will to live is controllable. It is when someone expects to be withdrawn, isolated, and useless, after a certain age—they create the very conditions that justify their belief. Our deepest assumptions are the triggers for physical changes."

Women should consider his theory seriously. It can change one's approach to aging, as it did mine. After reading his book, I feel Deepak Chopra has changed the aging process from a perceived threat to a desirable goal.

> *"We are made victims of sickness, aging, and death—by our fearful images of growing old: A self-fulfilling expectation of inevitable decline, and increasing feebleness in mind and body."*
>
> DEEPAK CHOPRA

According to Deepak Chopra, "aging seems to be something that's happening to you, when in fact it is something your body has largely learned to do. It has learned to carry out the programming fed into it by you—the programmer. Much of this programming is unconscious, dictated by beliefs and assumptions you hardly knew you held." He continues to explain that the number of impressions that get laid down inside us is staggering. Behavioral psychologists have estimated that just the verbal cues fed to us by our parents in early childhood, which still run inside our heads like muffled tape loops, amount to over 25,000 hours of pure conditioning.

It is this conditioning that has created our inherited expectation that the body must deteriorate over time. Combine that expectation with a deep belief that we are fated to suffer, grow old, and die, and you create, according to Deepak Chopra, "the biological phenomenon we call aging."

Our notions of aging have been dramatically modified over the last two decades. In the early 1970s doctors began to notice that some people in their sixties and seventies had bodies

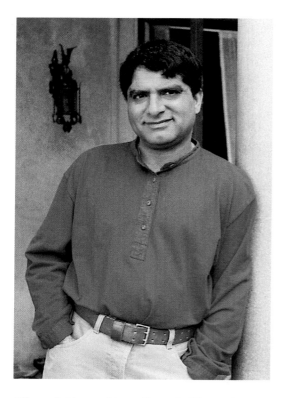

Through his teachings, Deepak Chopra has profoundly influenced my life.

deteriorate; rather, it gets stronger. Leg bones gain mass in proportion to how much weight is put on them (thus the need for weight-bearing exercise), which is why osteoporosis is unknown in tribal societies where life-long physical activity is the norm."

But though we may have this negative cultural expectation of aging, there are also signs of true progress. "Women in their fifties and sixties have the highest reported rates of mental health," says Ellen McGrath. Your sex life can also improve at this stage. Women report that the combination of freedom from birth control worries, increased self-confidence, and greater self-knowledge can lead to a greater enjoyment of sex, and Dr. McGrath confirms that experts now believe sex helps keep you healthy at any age.

And today, instead of feeling the empty nest syndrome and boredom, women in their fifties and sixties often feel what anthropologist Margaret Mead called "postmenopausal zest": a wonderfully intense joy in living. While they may feel temporarily depressed over particular problems, they can bounce back. They move into this later portion of their

that still functioned with the vigor and health of middle age. These people ate sensibly and looked after their bodies. Although it appeals to common sense that we grow old because we simply wear out, no wear-and-tear theory of aging has held up under close scrutiny. Deepak Chopra offers an excellent analogy: "A well exercised bicep doesn't

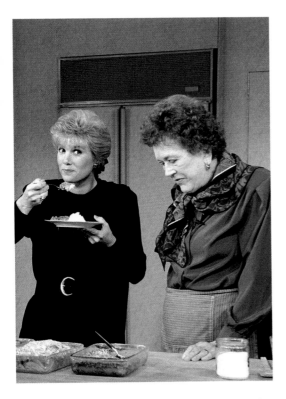

On the set of GMA with Julia Child, one of our favorite family members, still going strong in her eighties.

lives with incredible energy and focus.

One example is Barbara Johnson, Christopher Reeve's mom, who has taken up sculling (competitive rowing) at age sixty-four. Because of her chronic asthma, she had not actively participated in sports for most of her life. At an age when many of her contemporaries are backing away from challenges, competitive rowing has brought new focus and athleticism to her life.

Mrs. Johnson credits rowing for the current tide of happiness in her life. It has helped her manage her asthma better, given her a new physical confidence that she never had before, and helped her better cope with family crises without falling apart. Finding something that keeps you physically active as you get older will keep you sharp, healthy, and vivacious.

"Life itself is the proper binge."
JULIA CHILD

In *Ageless Body, Timeless Mind,* Deepak Chopra lists three ways to measure your age. I found his explanation extremely interesting, and think you will too.

1. *Chronological age*—how old you are by the calendar

2. *Biological age*—how old your body is in terms of critical life signs and cellular processes such as your pulse...

3. *Psychological age*—how old you feel you are

Only the first of these is fixed—yet chronological age is also the most unreliable gauge of the three. Biological age is changeable—regular physical exercise can reverse ten of the most typical effects of biological age, including high blood pressure, excess body fat, improper sugar balance, and decreased muscle mass. Accept better lifestyle habits, and you can improve your life expectancy on average by ten years. Thus the arrow of time can move forward quickly or slowly, stop in its tracks, or even turn around. Your body becomes younger or older biologically, depending on how you treat it.

Your third age—your psychological age—is even more flexible and is completely personal. A regular daily routine and being an optimist, as positive contributors to having a positive psychological age, whereas becoming self-absorbed is one of the most dangerous risks. Counting the times a person says "I" is a way to quantify self-absorption. A University of California psychologist, Larry Sherwitz, studied six hundred men suffering from heart disease. He counted how often each man used the words "I," "me," and "mine."

He found the men who used the first-person pronoun most often had the highest risk of heart trouble. And those who habitually talked about themselves {had} the greatest chance of a coronary. You need to listen with regard when others talk; give your time and energy to others; let others have their way; do things for reasons other than furthering your needs—and you will age well.

Assume, expect, and intend to remain at the most youthful level of functioning possible and intend to improve it every day. Do not set any restrictive expectations.

I saw a T-shirt recently that said, "Eat Right. Exercise. Die anyway." No question, our time on this earth is limited. But you can have a good deal of control over how long you'll live and how good you'll feel. We live in a time when planning ahead, eating right, strength training, and building muscle and bone mass is going to make a difference.

Daring gerontologists at Tufts University put a group of frail nursing home residents, ages eighty-seven to ninety-six, on a weight training regimen. Within eight weeks, wasted muscles had come back by

300 percent, coordination and balance improved, and overall, the people returned to a more active lifestyle. Some of these subjects had not been able to walk unaided but could now get up in the middle of the night and go to the bathroom by themselves, an act of reclaimed dignity that is by no means trivial. These results were always possible—when the residents began to believe they could change their bodies they were able to take actions to improve themselves physically and thus changed how they were "aging."

According to Dr. John Rowe, director of the MacArthur Foundation Consortium on Successful Aging, less than one-third of what happens to your mind and body as you age is genetically programmed. And the longer you live, the less influence heredity has! Researchers have found that the keys to a long, healthy, and fun old age (not coincidentally the focal messages of this book!) are: staying active, connected, and in control of your life. It's your future—be there to enjoy it!

Here are just a few examples from the latest MacArthur Foundation studies:

- Treadmill exercise increases a nerve-growth factor in your brain. (No wonder I love my treadmill so much!) In other words, exercise not only helps your bones and muscles but also keeps your brain charged up for action. Everything is connected.

- Older people who get out and exercise their brains—travel, read, take courses—don't show as great a mental decline as do their couch-potato counterparts. They may even keep improving.

- Having friends you can count on and having confidence in yourself can reduce stress and protect you from disease.

Now that I know I have a lot of influence over whether or not I lose my memory and sit stuck in the porch rocker, I'm starting to looking forward to that stage of my life. In thirty years, when you see that colorfully dressed, attractive old lady whiz past you on the jogging trail or riding path, take a second look, and wave. It might be me!

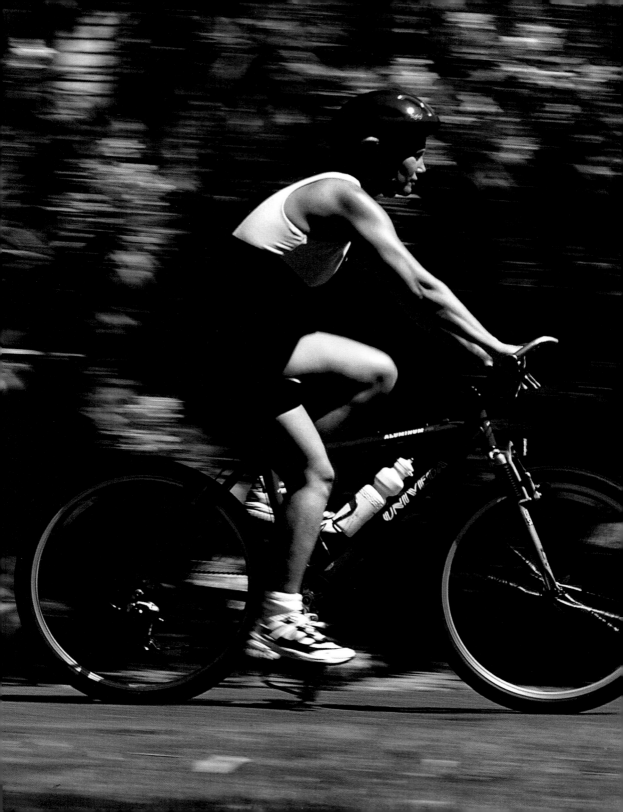

9 Honor Your Body

Life is like a ten-speed bike. We all have gears we never use.

—CHARLES SCHULZ

While perhaps the most important way to change your life is by changing the way you think and react, for total wellness, there is another half of the health equation: changing the way you care for your body. Remember, your mind and body are inextricably linked. This chapter will show you how to meet and conquer those daily demands that would otherwise sap your energy and stamina—and have some time left for yourself!

Eating for Healthy Living

Whether you're working long hours, raising a family, or training for an athletic competition, if you're going to be a winner you have to eat like one. "Poor nutrition practices contribute to every major health problem," says Dr. James M. Rippe. "Good nutritional patterns can play a crucial role in enhancing our health, happiness, and quality of life." To reap the benefits of a healthful diet, we need to learn those good practices, understand their importance, *and* put them to use.

I happen to be really lucky because I get to stay on top of the latest medical breakthroughs on a weekly basis through the *GMA* medical experts, Dr. Tim Johnson and Dr. Nancy Snyderman. They constantly remind all of us about our government's nutritional guidelines: eat a variety of foods, watch our fat intake, get regular physical activity, and maintain a healthy weight. They tell us to choose a diet low in fat, with plenty of vegetables and fruit, and to consume sugar, salt, and alcoholic beverages in

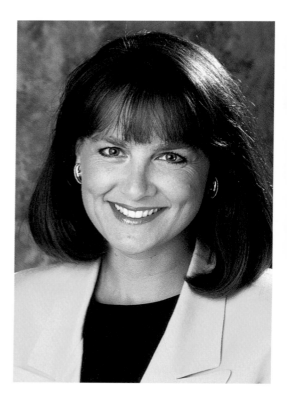

Dr. Nancy Snyderman.

moderation. Sounds easy, but when you're rushing off to work, eating whatever won't crumble or drip in the car, or cruising the cafeteria or the vending machines, it gets a lot more complicated. But once you've learned the ground rules they will become second nature, and eating healthily can become an integral and painless part of your lifestyle.

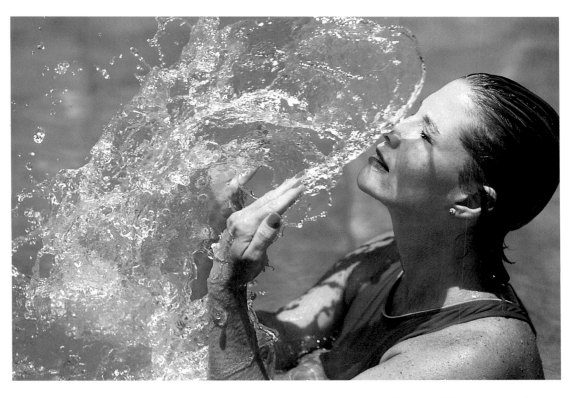

Water: The Secret Ingredient of Good Health

While you may not consider water a nutrient, it's actually the most critical one in your diet. Okay, let's face it: many of us think there's nothing more boring than a plain ol' glass of water. But water serves a greater purpose than simply quenching your thirst. Did you know that blood is 85 percent water and that

water also makes up 75 percent of your brain and 70 percent of your muscles? Water is behind all kinds of essential functions: it keeps you cool, helps you digest food, lubricates your joints, cushions your insides, and washes out wastes.

Even if you spend more time in the lounge chair than on the tennis court, you're still losing enough water each day to fill eight or ten glasses. Water sneaks out of your system without you noticing; you lose some just by breathing out.

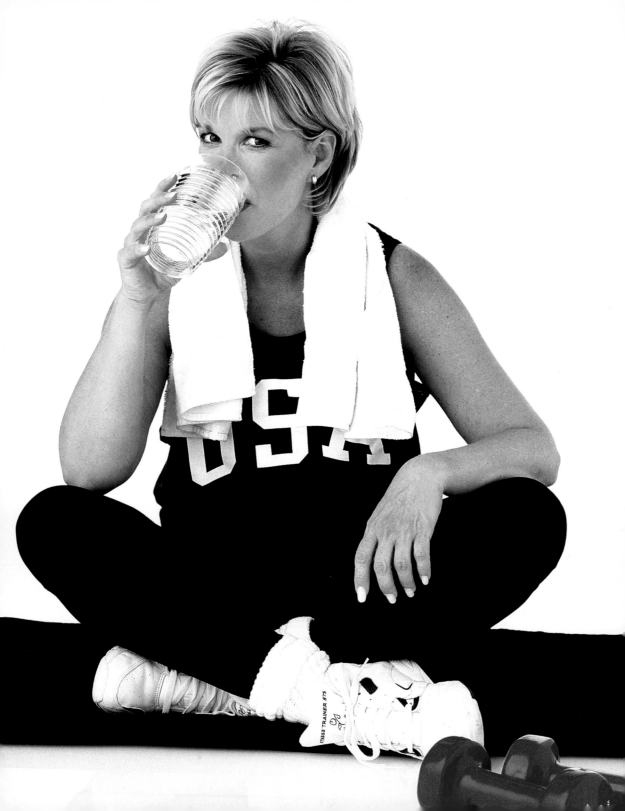

That's why you hear so much about the "eight glasses a day" rule. That's eight to ten 8-ounce glasses, folks. Most of us drink less than half that much!

"A lot of people walk around in a state of chronic dehydration, and feel fatigue from that," explains Ellie Krieger, nutritionist on staff at La Palestra. "Then they drink coffee for a little boost—but coffee further dehydrates you."

You may need even more than eight glasses a day, depending on what you're doing and where you are. If you live in a warm or dry climate or at a high altitude, or if you breathe dry air from a heater, dehumidifier, or air conditioner, your fluid loss increases dramatically. Plane travel also induces water loss: during a three-hour flight, you can actually lose one-and-a-half pints of water. Even a sunburn can increase water loss.

One way to tell if you're drinking enough is to do a quick check when you visit the bathroom. Lots of pale yellow urine is good; small amounts of dark urine mean more trips to the water fountain are in order. If you're pregnant or breast-feeding, or if you're postmeno-

Drink water before, during, and after exercise.

pausal, it's especially important to tote that water bottle. If you have kids along, be sure to share; they need extra water, too.

Water and Exercise

When you exercise, you lose an enormous amount of water, which must be replaced. Athletes don't carry around water just for show. An hour of working out can easily cost you one to two quarts of water, doubling your daily water need.

Even when you're not exercising, waiting to drink until you're thirsty is like waiting to gas up your car until the needle is on the big red E. According to Susan Kalish, executive director of the American Running and Fitness Association, by the time you feel thirsty, you're already dehydrated. Don't wait— hydrate yourself continually.

Losing just 2 percent of your body's water hurts your exercise performance. When I started to exercise seriously, I learned very quickly that if I didn't keep a water bottle near my treadmill, I tired much faster and even felt a little dizzy.

Here are some easy steps to help keep you hydrated throughout your workout:

1. *Drink before you exercise.* To make up for the inevitable sweat loss, drink two glasses of water at least a half hour before your workout.

2. *Drink frequently during your workout.* Remember that water bottle.

3. *Drink cool fluids.* This helps keep you cool. Despite the myths, cool fluids will not cause cramping.

4. *Drink after exercise.* Your sensation of thirst doesn't always reflect your real need for water. Drink two or three glasses *after* you've quenched your thirst.

The Skinny on Fat

A low-fat diet is the way to go for lower weight and better health. Our government says fat should make up no more than 30 percent of our total diet, but the average American eats more than that, and some of us eat a lot more. Overall, this is good advice for both health and energy.

"Fat takes longer to digest than protein or carbohydrates," says registered dieti-

tian Michelle Daum. "That's why, when you eat a fatty meal, you feel full, satisfied —yet tired and sluggish. If Americans could cut down on the ground beef, whole milk, cheese, lunch meats, and buttery desserts and reduce the amount of *saturated* fat they consume to 9 percent, about 100,000 first heart attacks could be prevented by the year 2005!"

However, when we try to put this advice into practice, some of us start worrying about the wrong things and end up worse off than we started.

The no-fat frenzy is why reduced-fat and fat-free cookies have beaten out Oreos as the number one cookie in America. "People got the message to reduce fat," says Dr. James M. Rippe, "but what they forgot was that if they eat foods that are laden with sugar instead of fat, they will still gain weight."

"Everybody's gotten fooled, because fat-free is not calorie-free," says Daum. "They thought as long as it was fat-free, they could eat as much as they wanted. They just went berserk. And they didn't lose weight, and they felt betrayed." There may be no fat in these new cookies, but they still have as many calories as an Oreo. Maybe that's why Americans on the whole are actually fatter than we were when the no-fat craze started! "My most important advice is to practice moderation," Daum says. "Don't go crazy buying all this fat-free stuff. You can lower your fat intake and still be overweight, which means you're at just as much risk for health problems as you were when you were consuming a high-fat diet!"

Sneaky Ways to Cut Down on Fat

One way to decrease the fat in your diet is to use the shrink-and-surround strategy: take a smaller portion of your favorite high-fat food—say, steak—and surround it with bigger portions of low-fat foods such as steamed vegetables and rice.

Try using less of the fatty food you really love and substituting low-fat foods for others. Use less butter or margarine on your bread and less mayonnaise in your tuna fish, or put mustard on your sandwich instead. Have a fruit sorbet or nonfat frozen yogurt instead of ice cream.

Another trick is to eat more high-fiber foods. Fiber not only leaves less room for fatty foods but helps push fat through your system faster, so you absorb less of it. But be careful: bran muffins, for example, are a source of high fiber, but they're not always low in calories. As a source of fiber you might prefer extra fresh fruits and vegetables, which are naturally low in calories and fat, or you could try a low-fat bran cereal.

The National Cancer Institute is rooting for us all to eat five servings of fruits and veggies a day. That seems easy, right? But surveys have found that on an average day, over 40 percent of us do not eat even *one* serving. A lot of room for improvement there. And what a difference something so simple could make!

Carbs vs. Proteins: A Heated Debate

Because many people are feeling let down by the fat-free approach to weight loss, we're seeing a new interest in protein-heavy diets. But many experts advise caution. "I don't endorse these diets," says Michelle Daum. "One of the things that's particularly unhealthy about them is that they're very low in carbohydrates. That's not healthy for the body or the brain." Another problem is that a high-protein diet leads to diet-and-binge cycles, since any diet that excludes basic food groups isn't healthy for the long run.

"There's almost nothing bad to say about carbohydrates," says Dr. James Rippe—especially the complex carbos we get from fruit and vegetables, beans, and whole grain pasta, breads, cereal, and rice.

"Dairy gets sort of a big, bad reputation," fitness expert Pat Manocchia has told me. "It's actually a great source of protein. Nonfat milk and yogurt are great, absolutely. And a piece of cheese occasionally is not going to kill you." And with those dairy products, you get a big dose of calcium. (More later about how important that is.)

The Sinister S-Words: Salt and Sugar

I've always craved salty snack foods, but I have always worked hard to cut down on my salt intake. What are the experts saying now?

"I think that the average person who has normal blood pressure does not need to worry very much about salt in her diet," says Dr. Rippe. "There's even a debate about whether people who have high blood pressure need to worry about salt." *Now* they tell me!

But hold on, it's not all good news. New research has confirmed that the more salt you eat, the more calcium you lose from your body—and the more likely you are to break bones when you're older. If you eat less sodium (table salt is 40 percent sodium), you'll keep more bone density, but you should make sure to include lots of calcium-rich foods in your diet and even take calcium supplements if your doctor recommends them. Also remember that some people are sensitive to sodium, which causes their bodies to retain water, making them look and feel bloated.

To cut down on salt without missing it too much, Michelle suggests that we substitute more homemade meals for the packaged stuff: "That includes canned soup, frozen dinners, Rice-A-

Roni, and Hamburger Helper. All of these foods contain very, very high levels of salt or sodium." And Dr. Rippe adds, "The more fresh products you eat —grains, fresh produce, fruits, vegetables, that sort of thing—the less salt you'll have in your diet." Daily sodium intake should not exceed 2,000 milligrams. Avoid salt substitutes, and use herbs and spices instead.

Okay, what about the other S-word: sugar? By itself, sugar isn't evil. But "sugar contributes in a major way to obesity and in a major way to tooth decay, which is also something that we tend to not think about," says Dr. Rippe.

Sugar is a nutritional zero. It fills you up (and out), is loaded with calories, and has no nutritional value. Still, sweet foods, especially chocolate, are the ones women most often crave. I've found it helpful to look at what sensation or taste I'm craving. Do I want something sweet, salty, or crunchy? Then I look for a calorie-reasonable alternative to fulfill that taste I'm seeking. If you're in the mood for something crunchy, for example, there are plenty of healthy and nutritious cereals that you can snack on, or try pretzels,

which are usually fat-free. You just have to become a label reader.

Recognizing the actual effects that certain foods have on my body has helped me better understand how to avoid or combat their consequences. For example, I know that if I eat a lot of salty foods, I can weigh as much as five extra pounds, because my body will retain water. My daughter Lindsay found that cutting way back on her sugar intake reduced her frequent headaches. If you pay attention to the effects foods have on *you,* you might be surprised at how even slight adjustments to your diet can make a dramatic difference in how you feel.

Peak Energy Foods

Whether you're preparing for a record-breaking run or just running for the bus, in today's nonstop world you need to have enough energy to get moving and to keep going full-tilt. That's why one of my favorite books lately is *Power Foods* by Liz Applegate. Power foods energize you for a demanding day and speed your recovery afterward.

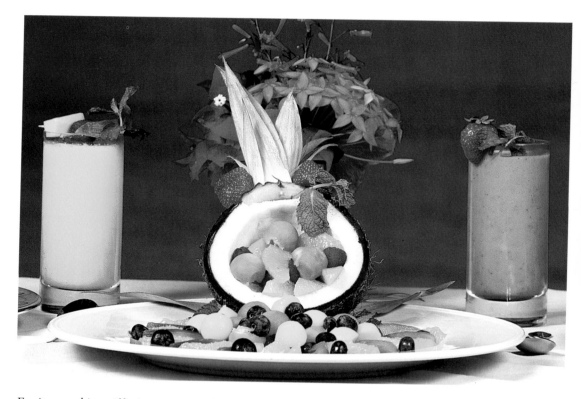

Fruit smoothies will give you a quick energy boost without too much fat or too many calories.

I asked Michelle Daum what else she recommends for those of us who need an occasional energy boost. Here are some of her favorite quick pick-me-up foods:

◆ Fruit Smoothie (see opposite page)
◆ A bowl of fresh fruit, including orange slices and berries
◆ Melon half filled with blueberries, which also has great eye-appeal, perhaps with a slice of seven-grain bread
◆ All kinds of dried fruits. Dried fruits can be fattening in large quantities, though, so moderate your intake. Remember, two dried apricot halves equal a whole fresh apricot.
◆ Sesame breadsticks
◆ Baked corn chips with salsa
◆ A mini-bagel
◆ Cheerios with raisins

FRUIT SMOOTHIE

MAKES 1 GENEROUS DRINK

1 cup plain, low-fat yogurt
  (see Note)
2 bananas (must be ripe)
8 medium strawberries,
  stemmed

1 cup crushed ice
Approximately 2 teaspoons
  honey

Blend together the yogurt, bananas, strawberries, ice, and honey in a blender. Depending on the sweetness of the bananas and strawberries, you may want to use a little more or a little less honey. Enjoy!

NOTE: Vanilla yogurt makes a tasty substitution for plain yogurt. If you make this change, leave out the honey.

- Nonfat pretzels
- Gazpacho
- Cucumber raita with pita bread
- Yogurt with low-fat granola or Grape-Nuts cereal
- Trail mix
- A low-fat breakfast bar
- Graham crackers
- Fat-free Fig Newtons
- Raw vegetables with low-fat Italian dressing
- Frozen fruit juice bars

"If you don't have time for something fancy, grab some quick energy from a bagel and a banana or some apples and figs. If you're just eating fruit for energy, you need to eat pretty frequently," says dietitian Ellie Krieger. "It will give you a quick burst of energy, but also quickly dissipate." While these foods are nutritious, they do still contain calories, so don't overeat.

When you have a busy day and need longer-term energy, go for a substantial

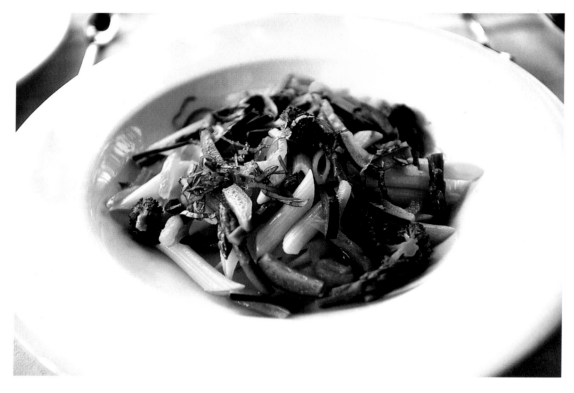

Penne pasta with vegetables will give you a long-term energy boost.

midday meal centered on complex carbs like whole-grain bread or pasta. Here are some ideas:

- Penne pasta with broccoli or asparagus
- Ratatouille
- Steamed vegetables with rice
- Pasta fagioli soup

- Grilled vegetables with couscous salad
- Minestrone-type soup with lots of veggies and pasta in it, and a piece of crusty bread
- Couscous salad with small currants and strips of red and yellow peppers
- A turkey sandwich with sprouts, honey mustard, and tomato on whole wheat bread
- White bean and vegetable soup
- Corn and potato chowder

- Sesame noodles with grilled chicken
- Chicken and vegetable kebabs over brown rice
- Black bean or vegetarian chili
- Pasta salad with sun-dried tomatoes and low-fat mozzarella
- Baked zucchini halves stuffed with fresh tomatoes or a mixture of roasted chicken, potatoes, and vegetables
- Vegetable lasagne made with low-fat cheese
- Spaghetti with Italian herbs
- Lentil salad with grilled vegetables
- Pita pizza with tomato and basil
- Orzo salad with raisins and sunflower seeds
- Vegetable stir-fry over brown rice
- Vegetable fajitas

Along with the carbohydrates, adds Krieger, "If you add a protein food, like turkey, beans, tofu, or nuts, that will help sustain you longer. For energy, the goal is to keep your blood glucose stable. Protein foods kick in after the complex carbohydrate foods, so [that combination] makes for a more even glucose level throughout the day." In plain old English, while protein may take a little longer than carbohydrates to boost your energy, the effect lasts longer.

Another way to boost your energy is to eat smaller amounts of food more often. Skipping meals, especially breakfast or lunch, is a major energy buster. "The rule of thumb is not to go more than five hours without eating something," says Ellie Krieger. If you get too hungry, you'll be tempted to pig out when you do sit down to eat.

What about the days when you're working out? "You should always eat something before you exercise, because your blood sugar may drop—but not directly prior to exercise," says Pat Manocchia. "A piece of fruit might be very good, because it's easily digested, or some carbohydrate, like a bagel. Avoid high-fat foods; don't have steak or a burger."

If you need extra energy for a hike or other longer effort, Pat recommends trail mix or gorp: good ol' raisins and peanuts. For long-distance runs or other demanding efforts, take along sports drinks, energy bars, or the new energy gels. Aim for 30 to 60 grams of carbs per hour—the amount in 24 ounces of sports drink, one energy bar, or two packets of energy gel.

The Benefits of Exercise

I know you're looking at this section and saying to yourself, "Exercise: that's getting on a treadmill and sweating. That's boring, and I don't have the time." Let's get this straight up front: exercise isn't about suffering; exercise is about finding something you enjoy doing that also happens to protect your health, lift your mood, and give your energy level a kick in the butt.

If you're in your twenties and finishing school, starting a career, and perhaps looking for a mate, exercise is something you do for cosmetic reasons, to look good. You probably aren't thinking of it in terms of preventing heart disease and osteoporosis—your forties seem aeons away!

By the time you're into your thirties and perhaps juggling the demands of spouse, kids, and job, "You start to realize that exercise has emotional benefits as well as physical benefits," says Barbara Brandt." It's at this time that many women start to reassess why they're exercising."

When you get into your forties, "Now you're hearing about osteoporosis," Bar-

bara notes. "You have a friend who just had a mastectomy. So-and-so's friend died of heart disease. All of a sudden the statistics you've always heard about—that you thought were so many years away from you—come into serious consideration."

"After menopause, heart disease is six to ten times more likely to kill a woman than breast cancer. After heart disease, everything else is a distant second, third, and fourth," says Dr. James Rippe. Of course, that doesn't mean cancer isn't scary and that you shouldn't do breast self-exams and get your mammograms. However, we do know a lot about preventing heart disease today—and exercise is the key.

New research shows that if you can add just an extra thirty minutes of moderate activity to your everyday routines, you'll get a significant health payoff. So park a few blocks away from the office and walk in. Jog a bit with the dog. Take the stairs instead of the elevator. Ride an exercise bike while you watch

Barbara Brandt and me in a photograph taken for the cover of my exercise video, Workout America.

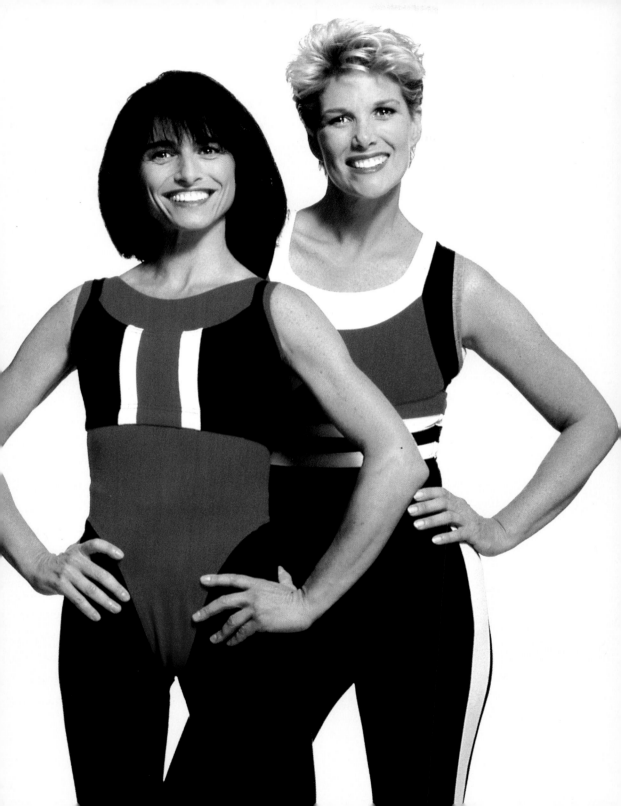

your favorite TV show. You'd be surprised at how fast you can accumulate that thirty minutes—and you thought you weren't an exercise person!

Exercise for a Good Mental Attitude

While improving your health is the primary reason for exercise, it also helps you feel better about yourself. And I don't just mean feeling good about the way you look.

Barbara Brandt was the person who got me started on this path.

When Joan started training with me, she was working on the tangible: looking at the scale and saying, "Am I a good girl today or a bad girl? Am I worthy? Do I deserve?" Joan was going back out into the single world, and felt she needed to feel good about herself. Everybody wants to look good, to feel comfortable tucking in her T-shirt.

I remember the time when she finally realized that there was so much more to

exercise than seeing the numbers on the scale move down. Joan was going through her divorce and sometimes she would be upset. She knew that a strategy for her emotional well-being was getting on the treadmill. She knew that when she'd get on the treadmill, she'd feel like one person, and when she'd get off she'd feel like another.

Here's a person who had little time to sleep. And I can't tell you the number of times she called me or reported to me the next day and said, "You know, I really should have been in bed. But I knew I wasn't going to fall asleep. I was too stressed out. I went down and I did an hour on the treadmill. I went to bed feeling like a new person."

Ironically, it was by getting serious about exercise that I was able to get off my emotional treadmill and stop being so self-critical. While looking good in jeans is terrific, it's the reduced stress, increased energy, and feeling of accomplishment I get from exercise that will really do the job.

"I've worked with a lot of people and I have never seen anybody satisfied with an aesthetic goal," says Pat Manocchia.

"Once a certain body part shrinks, they want to make another one bigger. However, if someone can actually do something they've never been able to do before their whole self image seems to change. Accomplishment is the best form of motivation. Ultimately you have to decide how you feel about yourself based on who you are inside, not because of a number on the scale.

"It's my belief that exercise can have a positive influence on all the other things in your life," says Pat, "and exercise is one factor that's very tangible and controllable. You can't really affect one part of your life without affecting the others in some way. And exercise makes people's lives better." says Pat. I guess that's why Pat made a career choice to help people reach their fitness goals and to improve their overall health and well-being.

Ways to Get Moving

What was that you said about not having time for exercise? "I've heard that before," says Pat Manocchia. "I've worked with some people who were extremely busy, with very, very high-demand schedules. What I usually tell them is 'Look, the president of the United States exercises four times a week. If you can tell me you're busier than the president, then I'll believe you!'"

Here is Barbara Brandt's advice for fitting in exercise:

Many of my clients are working women who take 6:00 A.M. trains and get home at 8:00 in the evening. They walk in, and they're bombarded with kids, and a husband they haven't seen all day.

My recommendation to them is to get up earlier! I know it sounds like a complete impossibility, but the thirty or forty-five minutes' worth of exercise is much more valuable than the extra minutes of sleep.

I'll say, okay, instead of penciling in exercise, we're going to put it in ink. And you're going to write into your calendar three or four days' worth of exercise this week: walking on the treadmill, taking a walk outside, putting on a videotape and exercising with the TV, or whatever works for

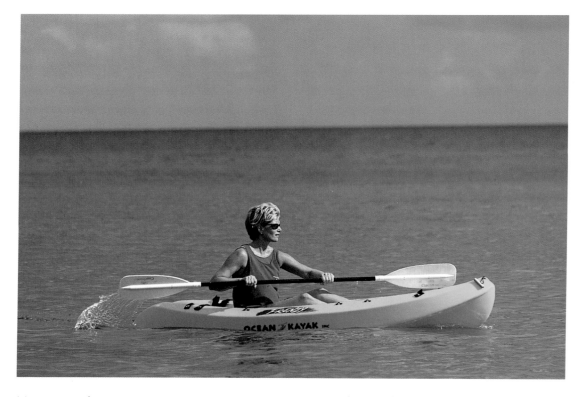

Trying something new.

you. And then we'll do it again for week two, three, and four.

At the end of the month, you're going to assess it. Look back and say, "Do I feel sleep-deprived, or do I feel more physically fit and clear-headed? Am I less stressed out and a better mother and wife because I'm getting a lot of stuff out of my system by exercising?"

Of the hundreds of people I've

worked with over the years, I have yet to have one person come up to me and say, "You know, this really wasn't a good strategy. Do you have something else you can give me?"

Barbara also recommends lunch-hour mall-walking, especially if you live in a steamy or snowy climate. It helps to get a fitness buddy: you're less likely to bail out, and you get a chance to socialize.

Realize that exercise doesn't always

require a gym. It doesn't always require special clothing or removing your makeup. You can get down on the floor and exercise while you watch the news.

Barbara says, "If I find that I'm short on time and my child needs help with homework, I'll say, 'Bring your homework upstairs, and let's do it while I'm on the treadmill'" There are *always* ways of fitting it in.

What Are Your Exercise Goals?

Pat Manocchia stresses the importance of starting out with your goals clearly in mind.

Goals first and foremost must be realistic. And to meet them, you need some sort of a map. If you haven't been working out on a regular basis, start with simple goals that you'll achieve, so that you won't get frustrated and give up. If you've been working out but need a goal, find something to train for that interests you, like a charity run or, like Joan did, a mountain

climb. The important thing to remember is to have a purpose and stick with it. The results will simply follow.

See your doctor for a physical check-up before you start any exercise program, especially if you haven't moved around much for a while.

An important part of setting your goals is realizing that a realistic exercise plan is not another fad program that you go on and off within a few weeks. We're talking about a new way of life for the rest of your life. Say to yourself, "I'm going to take good care of myself. I need it, and I deserve it." Now say it out loud!

Once you're under way with your exercise plan, you need to add some variety to it so you won't get bored. There are a lot of fun physical things to try in the world. Why not find out all that your body can do? Try something different, like windsurfing, in-line skating, or boxing.

"If you have a hard time doing it, get some help," says Pat Manocchia. "Because if you exercise properly, it's the fairest court in the land. If you put in the work and you put in the time and you do it properly, you will see a result every single time," he says. "There is no other place in the world in your life that you will experience that fairness. In relationships, in your job, you can do all the work, work hard, and still not see a result. That will not happen with your body. If you do it, you will see the result."

Maximize Efficiency

One of my top priorities when I began exercising, since my schedule is so tight, was figuring out how to get the most benefit from the amount of time I put in. I started out doing dumb things, like skimping on stretching. I wanted to burn more calories! I soon figured out that you pay a big price in pain and stiffness if you don't stretch, and you may be too sore to exercise the next time. Experts say that the secret to exercising efficiently is to know what you're doing. That's why it's so important to work with a class, a trainer, or a video when you start.

I'm a very driven person. Once I com-

mitted myself to exercising, I wanted to go all out and *see some results!* But I finally got it through my head that exercising seven days a week accomplishes less than working out four days does. Resting is sometimes called the other half of the workout. It's during rest and recovery that you actually *get* the results as your body responds to the stress you've put on it. If you can't stand to sit still, try "active rest": doing something like walking, that keeps you moving but is easier on your body than your regular workout.

So what is the right amount of exercise? To get what's called the aerobic training effect—a stronger heart that can pump more blood, and muscles that can make better use of the oxygen they get—you can follow a number of general guidelines. For example, the American College of Sports Medicine suggests three to five aerobic exercise sessions each week, with each session lasting fifteen to sixty minutes, supplemented by a strength training program.

Experts now believe that for the average person who's not an elite athlete in training, accumulated time is just as good as condensed time. That means if it's hard for you to put in sixty minutes three times a week, go for six thirty-minute workouts.

Is it better still if you put in four sixty-minute sessions a week? If you're training on a deadline—say, for a marathon or a mountain climb—it's probably worth it. For the ordinary exerciser, when you're looking for results over six months or a year, "The results will be the same—they'll just take longer to accumulate," says Pat Manocchia. He is well aware of our culture's desire for immediate gratification:

Unfortunately . . . we're time-fixated. We want it now! People come to me and say, "I have to shoot a movie in four weeks. What can I do?" Well, nothing. What we want to do is make fitness a lifestyle.

It depends on where you start. But for the average person, making that lifestyle change takes six months, minimum.

I had a guy come to me who was a very successful businessman, very motivated. He said, "I have to come in five times a week. I really want it!" I said, "No, you can't. You have

to come in three times a week."

Why? I knew that ultimately this guy would end up averaging four times a week, but because he'd wanted to come in five times a week, he would feel defeated. He'd feel that he didn't accomplish his goal. He would have been depressed, and after six months he would have stopped coming. If he does it three times a week, he'll see the results—and see them relatively quickly—and he'll be much more likely to stay with it. The idea is to make activity part of your life.

Target Heart Rate

How do you know your heart is pumping hard enough to get stronger but not so hard that you're overdoing it? That's where knowing your target heart rate can help. Your target heart rate is a range, or a window, that indicates whether you're working your body efficiently.

So how do you determine your appropriate workout level? Well, your target heart rate depends on your age and your fitness goals. "If your goal is simply to lower your risk of chronic disease, there is no reason to exercise at more than 50 to 60 percent of your target heart rate," says James Rippe. "If your goal is weight management, our recommendation is 60 to 80 percent of your predicted maximum heart rate." The bottom line here: if you want to burn fat and reduce calories, you must figure out what your maximum efficiency range is and stay within it during your workout.

HERE'S HOW TO FIND YOUR TARGET (ESTIMATED) RANGE:

1. Estimate your maximum heart rate by subtracting your age from 220. If you're forty-five, your maximum heart rate is 175 beats per minute. That's the absolute ceiling.

2. Find your training heart rate. For the most effective aerobic workout, you must train between 60 and 80 percent of your maximum heart rate. To find the rate you want, multiply each percentage

TARGET HEART RATE FINDER

Workout Range		Effective Aerobic	
Your Age	Max Heart Rate	60% of Max	80% of Max
20 years	200 beats/min.	120 bpm (20 per 10 secs)	160 bpm (26)
30	190	114 (19)	152 (25)
40	180	108 (18)	144 (24)
50	170	102 (17)	136 (23)
60	160	96 (16)	128 (22)
70	150	90 (15)	120 (20)

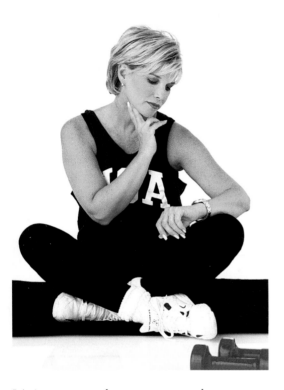

It's important to know your target heart rate so you get the most benefits from your workout.

rate by six: 105/6 = 17.5 —140/6 = 23.3. Your range is 17 to 23 beats every ten seconds. Take your pulse for ten seconds during exercise. If you're working within your target heart rate range, 17 to 23 beats every ten seconds will indicate effective aerobic training. If your pulse rate is below the lowest number, you must work harder to be effective. If it's higher, you are working out at a dangerous level and must reduce the level of intensity.

Increase Your Metabolism with Weight Training

times your maximum heart rate. If you're forty-five and want to train at 60 to 80 percent of your maximum rate, then .60 x 175 = 105 heartbeats per minute. This is the low end of your training range, and .80 x 175 = 140 bpm, which is the high end.

3. To calculate your range while working out, divide your training heart

When you hear the words "muscle mass," do you think, Yecch! I don't want huge muscles! Don't worry. "Women, first of all, don't have the hormonal material in them to make themselves very big," Pat Manocchia points out. "You'd have to do a significant amount of lifting: very heavy weights, for a couple of hours, almost daily."

Actually, a reasonable amount of muscle makes you look slimmer. "A pound of muscle is about as big as a baseball or

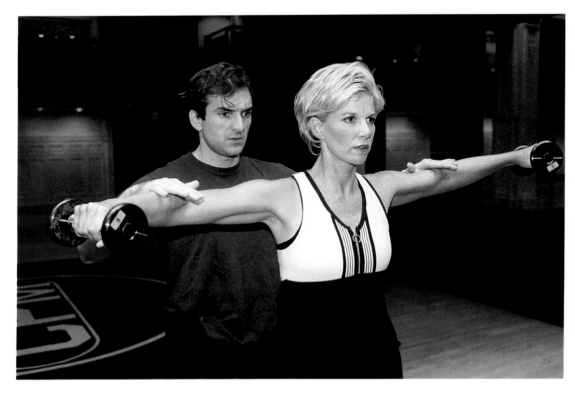

ABOVE: *Training with Pat Manocchia.*
OPPOSITE: *Weight training has increased my strength and given my body more definition.*

orange; a pound of fat's about as big as a softball or a grapefruit," says Pat. "One person can weigh 130 pounds and have a 32-inch waist, while another can weigh the same and have a 28-inch waist. The person with the 28-inch waist would have more muscle."

Muscle is also a bigger calorie burner.

According to Dr. James Rippe, "The higher the muscle mass you carry through your life, the more likely it is that you're going to be able to control your weight. Lots of people have been able to control their weight simply by running or jogging. And if they then start strength training, they can get a dramatic boost in their metabolism because they've increased their lean muscle mass." This means that if you have more muscle, you can eat more and gain less weight!

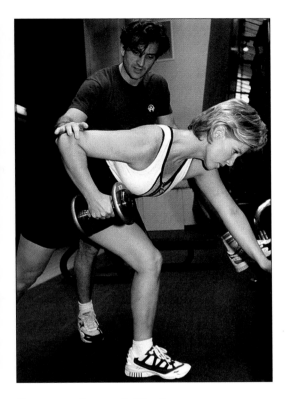

Strength and Endurance Training

While aerobic fitness used to get all the press, we're starting to hear more about the health benefits of muscular fitness Translation: it's not just for body-builders anymore! Besides the extra help with fat burning, strength training increases your ability to get things done in day-to-day life—what experts call functional fitness—and to keep on doing those things for years longer.

Because we're so obsessed with our hips, butt, and thighs, a lot of us neglect to work our upper bodies. Maybe it's also because leg work is easier and upper body work is hard. It's natural to prefer to do things you're good at doing. But as Barbara and Pat have taught me, balance is everything: in exercise, in eating, in everything you do.

"We did upper body work with Joan because she needed to develop joint integrity in her shoulders and back, develop postural muscles, and basically become stronger," says Pat.

"When she went mountain-climbing, she'd have to carry a big pack on her back. She'd have to be able to stop herself if she fell, and she needed strength in order to do that."

Working out has had many benefits in my life. The emotional benefits have been terrific, especially in terms of providing me with a more positive self-image. I look better and, in case you hadn't noticed, I definitely feel better about myself. One of the most surprising effects that working out has had on my body came, well, you might say as a

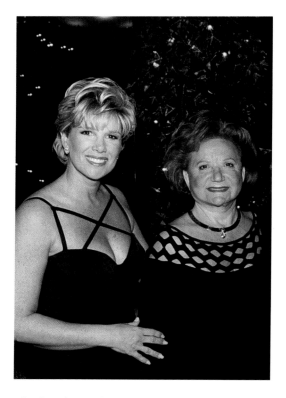

If only I had inherited my mother's D cups, I wouldn't have had to lift all those weights!

I worked out like crazy, and it was finally the evening of the big event. I slid that dress up my body, zipped it up, did one final check in the mirror, and was out the door. I felt that I looked the best I had in years.

I mingled during the hors d'oeuvres, greeting many dear old friends whom I hadn't seen for ages. From across the room I saw my former personal assistant of eight years, Debbie Bergenfeld-Bierman. She came like a bullet across the room, screaming, "OH, MY GOD! WHEN DID YOU GET A BOOB JOB?"

I was shocked by her comment, but the surprised look on my face was no help as I denied her allegation. It's so funny, because this is a woman who saw me in my clothes, out of my clothes, pregnant, heavy, and thin again. She knows my body almost as well as I do. After all, she was responsible for my wardrobe during those eight years and often helped me choose outfits to wear on the air and for personal appearances.

Suddenly I realized that it must be all of the upper body work I had been doing at the gym. I remember Pat telling me that my pectoral muscles were getting

complete surprise, albeit a pleasant one.

I had been working out with Pat Manocchia for about six months, with an intense focus on shaping my upper body. I concentrated specifically on my arms, pectoral muscles, chest, and back. I had a black-tie dinner to attend in a few weeks, and a slinky, sexy, strappy black gown to fit my new body into.

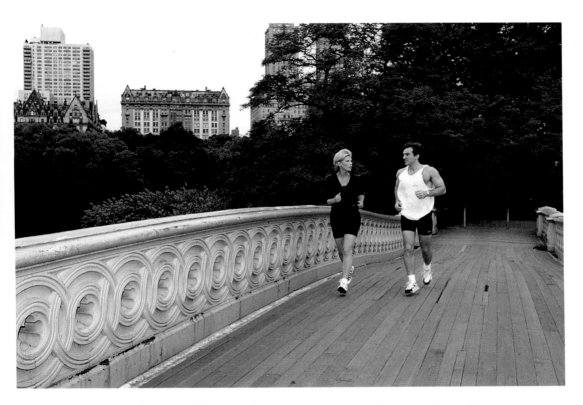

Running with Pat in Central Park.

nicely developed, but I didn't realize exactly what that meant in terms of my appearance until Debbie pointed it out, as only she could.

Debbie didn't want to believe that I was able to achieve such dramatic results through dedication, working out five days a week, and a lot of sweat! But it's the truth, and I was *finally* able to convince her. We had a good laugh over her absolute insistence that I must have had a boob job, and the fact that she was so hurt that I wouldn't tell her the truth.

Strength training is an area where you really need some guidance from a trainer or a video to make sure you're doing the exercises properly. It's easy to hurt yourself by overdoing it, or by training unevenly. (Sure, do those stomach crunches, but don't forget your lower back.)

Don't expect strength training to substitute for calorie burning. As Pat says,

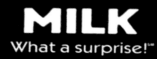

Most people think I must drink at least 10 cups of coffee to be so perky in the morning. But the truth is, I like skim milk first thing. It has all the same nutrients as whole milk without all the fat. And besides, my husband got the coffee maker.

MILK
What a surprise!℠

"Abdominal exercises are not going to make you lose body fat. They're not going to eliminate the roll around your tummy."

As for endurance, one way to build that fast is the way Pat taught me to prepare for my mountain climb: interval training. That means pushing yourself for a little, then slowing the pace, then picking it up again. I started by walking a half mile, running a quarter mile, then walking another half mile.

I had never liked running because I found it too hard. With interval training, I was amazed at how fast I was able to build my endurance to the point where I could comfortably run a half mile. To start, try just alternating walking and running every few minutes.

One of the great highs of exercise, for me, has been seeing myself accomplish things I never thought I'd even attempt. I like the way Pat Manocchia puts it:

I've seen people who are not in very good shape who have very good body images. Because they could accomplish something, they felt good about themselves. You can do it one step at a time. These people who climb the mountains and run the marathons are everyday, *normal people. They might have assumed that they never could do it, because they would never think of it. They'd just say, "Oh, that's for other people." That is, until they get into a system.*

All you have to do is take care of your body. Your body wants to be healthy. It doesn't want to be unhealthy. All you have to do is use it properly!

Building Better Bones: Preventing Osteoporosis

By age seventy-five, 90 percent of us are expected to have some osteoporosis. Osteoporosis can turn a simple twist or fall into a fractured wrist, spine, or hip. Just lifting a bag of groceries can be enough to crack a bone!

Although we picture them as cold and hard, bones are actually made of living cells, continually wearing out and building up again. For most of us, our bones are at their strongest—what experts call peak density—around our mid-thirties.

From there, your bones gradually lose cells, picking up speed in the first years after menopause, because less estrogen means faster bone breakdown. This is when you can lose 1 percent or more of your bone each year. And each 10 percent lost doubles your fracture risk!

The good news is that with a little information and planning, you can really improve your odds. There are simple and inexpensive things you can do now to build and keep stronger bones. Think of it as another way to save for retirement: you're building a bone-saving account to avoid a frail and fearful later life.

♦ *Eat calcium-rich foods.* Your body needs calcium to build those bones. "You need to have three or four servings a day of calcium-rich food," says Michelle Daum. "Dairy foods—milk, yogurt, and cheese—are the richest source of calcium; I recommend low-fat or nonfat dairy products."

There's also calcium in canned salmon, with bones, and sardines; in dried beans and peas, including cooked lentils, navy beans, and white beans; and in oranges, broccoli, and dark green leafy vegetables like spinach, kale, and mustard greens.

♦ *Take calcium supplements.* Most of us don't get enough calcium, even with a healthy diet. Doctors suggest stocking up on calcium pills and taking 1,000 milligrams a day—more if you're pregnant or postmenopausal.

♦ *Get enough exercise.* "The things that are important for women specifically to do over time are weight-bearing exercise and resistance training," says Pat Manocchia. "It can be weight training or push-ups or classes where you're on your feet or running—but something where you're bearing your weight."

If your bones are already on the fragile side, go for a low-impact weight-bearing workout. That might be a low-impact aerobics class, a walk in the woods, or stepping on a stair machine. Also get some balance and flexibility training, since it reduces your odds of falling.

And never assume it's too late for exercise. No matter what your age, it can make a real difference. A 1994 study published in the *Journal of the American Medical Association* found that seventy-year-olds who lifted weights twice a week not only prevented bone loss but actually added a bit more bone density!

◆ *Don't smoke, and drink only in moderation.* Whenever I hear that statement, I think of Dr. Tim Johnson, who has appeared on *GMA* many times to deliver this message. Each time, he looks me in the eye and says, "I know we've told them many times before, but maybe, just maybe, we'll save another life today." If you smoke, I'm sure you've heard a zillion reasons why you should quit. Here's reason one zillion and one: smoking decreases the estrogen circulating in your system and seems to make it harder to absorb calcium. Your bones don't need these problems. Having three or more drinks a day is also a bad idea, since alcohol interferes with the absorption of calcium and vitamin D.

◆ *Cut down on caffeine and some medicines.* Too much caffeine can cause problems with calcium. A 6-ounce cup of drip-brewed coffee has about 100 milligrams of caffeine; regular tea has about 50 mg; a 12-ounce glass of cola contains 36 mg.

Two or three cups of coffee a day probably won't hurt you. A cup or two can boost energy, concentration, and mood for the sleep-deprived. But when you get to four cups or so, the amount of caffeine you are consuming will block your body's absorption of calcium. And if you drink upward of half a dozen cups of coffee a day, take note: it may raise your cholesterol level and your risk of heart attack.

Bulk-forming laxatives like Metamucil also can interfere with calcium absorption; so can a diet very high in fiber (another plug for moderation in everything). Also watch out for medicines with hidden caffeine; there's a heaping helping of caffeine in some pain relievers, like Exedrin and Midol.

◆ *Consider taking medications.* Look at changing your health habits as your first line of defense, says Dr. Robert Recker, director of the Osteoporosis

Research Center in Omaha. Then, if you need to, add medications to your bone-defense arsenal.

In just the last year or two several new drugs have come out for women who already have weak bones. These include pills and nose sprays that can stop bone loss and cut your fracture risk by half. You can talk to a doctor about the pros and cons and about what your medical insurance will cover.

Estrogen is most often the first-choice drug to control osteoporosis. Women who start estrogen treatments after menopause get fewer fractures. Even if you're five or six years out from menopause, estrogen seems to help, and it doesn't cost all that much.

I've Got to Get Some Sleep!

Are we a nation of sleepy people? Well, research is showing that Americans are getting less and less sleep, and they're exhausted. Can a sleep-deprived country be efficient? A national commission set up to study the problem estimated that the cost of sleeplessness in accidents, low productivity, and illness was almost 16 billion dollars a year.

I interviewed Stanley Coren, author of *Sleep Thieves,* who says, "When you don't get enough sleep, it makes you clumsy, stupid, unhappy, and ultimately, dead."

We spend one-third of our lives sleeping, but we know very little about why we sleep. We do know it's important in repairing worn-out tissues, renewing brain structures, and releasing growth hormones. It's true: your kids really do grow overnight!

Stanley Coren says that "when you don't get enough sleep, one of the things that starts to happen is your ability to process information begins to stop. You actually act as though you're losing I.Q. points. In fact, if you lose an hour of sleep below eight hours, it's the equivalent of losing one point of I.Q." If you lose an hour below seven hours, you lose two points. And it adds up. So if you are losing two hours of sleep five days in a row, you've lost ten hours' worth of sleep—and fifteen points of I.Q. Being a person who suffers from constant sleep deprivation, I was anxious to ask if this loss was temporary or permanent—not that I was afraid of the answer or anything...I'm happy to say that it is, in fact, temporary. But that doesn't mean it's not dangerous. When we "spring ahead" for daylight savings time, that hour of lost sleep causes a 7 percent rise in traffic accidents that day!

How Much Sleep Do You Need?

Sleep needs change with age. If you have teenagers, you know that they can sleep for incredible lengths of time. At midlife, most people sleep about seven and a half hours a night. As you get older, it's normal to sleep fewer hours, take more naps, and wake up more often at night.

But tallying hours spent under the sheets isn't a good guide to whether you've had enough sleep. Some people feel great on six hours of rest; others really need ten. The question is, are you getting enough sleep to feel refreshed, alert, and not terminally cranky?

In a perfect world, we'd all sleep until we awaken by ourselves. Alarm clocks would go out the window, which is certainly where I'd like send mine most

mornings! But until that paradise arrives, here are some sleep suggestions:

- *Don't try to squeeze in exercise right before bed.* Give your muscles a rest from mid-evening on. Late afternoon exercise is probably ideal.

- *Skip the after-dinner cappuccino.* If you have caffeine two to four hours before bed, you'll probably toss and turn. Some people need to cut out coffee and all other caffeine products like chocolate, tea, and cola even earlier.

- *Watch what you eat at the end of the day.* A heavy evening meal, especially one that features spicy or gas-producing food, is also a recipe for poor sleep. The same goes for cigarettes and alcohol. You may think that alcohol makes you sleepy, but it actually disrupts your sleep.

- *Eat a "sleep snack."* Some experts believe that foods containing an amino acid (found in protein) called tryptophan can make you sleepy. Stanley Coren suggests that a glass of milk and a couple of aspirin might help if you're having sleep difficulties. I asked Michelle Daum for her take on this. "Tryptophan is a precursor for serotonin, which is a neurotransmitter that helps induce a feeling of sleepiness and calm," she explained. She recommends small amounts of starchy carbohydrates, low in protein and fat, consumed an hour or two before bedtime. Her favorites include:

- *pretzels*
- *breadsticks*
- *animal crackers*
- *dry nonsugary cereal*
- *toast*
- *an English muffin or a bagel*
- *baked bagel crisps*
- *rice cakes (not caramel)*
- *a low-fat toaster waffle*
- *oven-baked potato crisps*
- *graham crackers*
- *popcorn*
- *flatbreads*
- *a bowl of hot oatmeal*
- *plain biscotti*
- *baked corn-tortilla chips*

- *Give yourself an hour to relax* before you hit the hay. Develop a pre-sleep routine: listen to music, read, or take a warm (not hot) bath. Routines work for your kids—why not you?

- *Create a restful environment.* It's best to keep your bedroom a bit cool (60 to 65 degrees), dark, and quiet. Light and noise can affect the quality of your sleep even if they don't seem to wake you up. If you can't avoid them, try a sleeping mask and soft ear plugs.

- *Consider a better mattress.* If yours is too saggy, taut, or thin, it may be stealing your best sleep. When you shop for a new one, lie down for at least five minutes to see how it feels before you buy it. You deserve a decent introduction to something you'll cuddle up to eight hours a day.

- *Forget sleeping in.* You'll have more luck if you go to bed early than if you sleep late. By sleeping more than an hour past your usual wake-up time on the weekend, you can inadvertently reset your body clock and end up dragging on Monday morning. An early after-

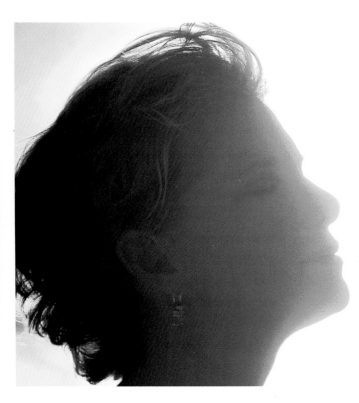

noon nap can also help you catch up—but keep it under an hour.

◆ *If you suffer from jet lag,* talk to your doctor about ways to prevent it with small doses of melatonin, a hormone that affects your body clock, or with timed exposure to bright lights.

◆ *If you can't fall asleep* after twenty minutes, get up. Read a dull book, or do relaxation exercises (see page 130). Go back to bed when you're sleepy. If you're not sleepy at all, don't get into bed. I often find that 20 minutes of meditation helps me get a full night's sleep.

If you honor your body, it will serve you well in return, in the present and for years to come. Getting started with healthy routines of diet, sleep, and exercise can be intimidating, but it's your body, it's your health, and you'll have yourself to thank!

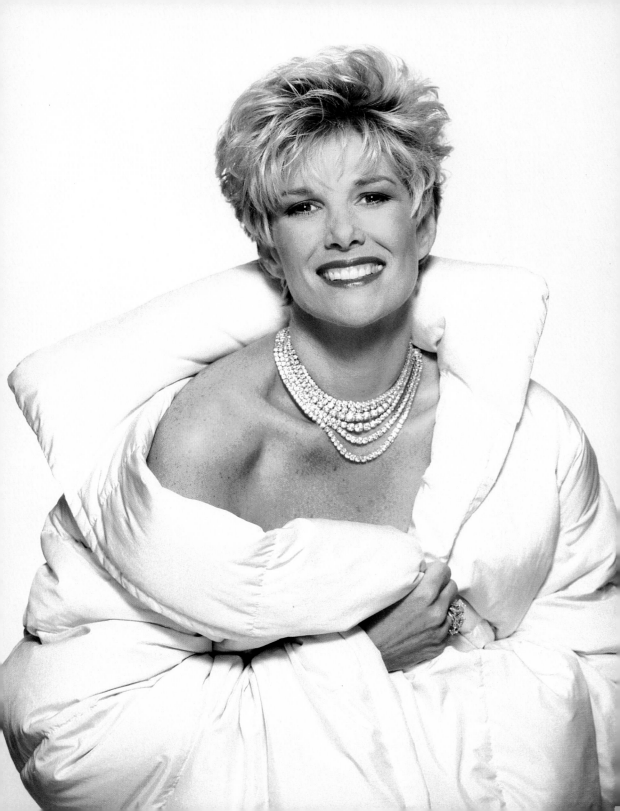

10 Change Yourself and Your Fortune Will Change

My life is much richer today because I have learned to look for the joy in each day. I am open to exploring new ideas and changing old habits. I am thankful for learning the importance of the continual search for inner peace. I hope that I will always be a work in progress, for that means that I will continue to grow, learn, and become a better person. I continue to learn to trust my instincts, I see that my needs are met, and therefore I will reach farther than I ever thought I could.

My life is rich because of the love that surrounds me through my family and my circle of close friends. I am learning to accept others for who they are and not for who I want them to be. I accept that I cannot change the world but that I can change myself. I now understand that forgiveness frees you of the anger that weighs you down and robs you of your energy. Gratitude—appreciating the love, joy, and contentment in my life—makes it much more meaningful.

My life is rich in its new calmness. Each day I live does not become a good or bad one because of what goes on around me but because of how I choose to deal with it. I am richer today for believing in myself, for that strength will carry me to higher peaks. It also gives me a voice, to better communicate with others. I am learning to be a better listener and to offer my support when it's needed.

I am also thankful that I found a healthy way of life, which ensures that I nurture my mind, body, and spirit. My new strength feeds my positive outlook. I feel I can now pass on to my girls this value of being confident and yet sensitive and caring to others.

Fortune has many definitions. I am always reminding my daughters to cherish and be thankful for all that they have. When I count my blessings, how could I not feel rich?

Oh, and by the way, the Donna Karan coat and the one million dollars' worth of Cartier diamonds I'm wearing in the last picture are not mine—only the sparkle in my eye and the joy in the smile on my face.

"Exude happiness—
and you will feel it back
a thousand times."

JOAN LUNDEN

Spas and Health Resorts

Spa-Finders is a specialized travel service that can help you find the right spa program to fit your needs and your budget. We use them whenever we go to a spa because they often can book accommodations at a better rate or with special perks that are only available through Spa-Finders. They can also provide additional information on the following spas, and others. For more than ten years, they have been publishing a directory of spas with hundreds of listings and detailed descriptions. The cost of the directory ($5.95) is refunded when you book your vacation with Spa-Finders. They also publish a quarterly roundup of special spa offers and discounted programs. Their travel service is free of charge, and their staff is helpful and knowledgeable about the various programs that are available. You can reach them by calling 800-255-7727, or in New York City, 212-924-6800.

Fitness, Beauty, and Wellness

Green Valley Spa
Utah

Beneath the clear blue skies of the Southwest desert, this southern Utah spa is surrounded by the beautiful red rock canyons and Zion National Park. It is a favorite among beginning and advanced hikers alike, and also offers exceptional tennis programs for any level of play. When your workout is finished, you can experience the sublime pleasure of exquisite spa treatments in the relaxation center. Trained specialists will help you determine your exact body type and then help you select the perfect diet, based on your tastes and your ability to metabolize foods. Exceptional healing therapists and weight-loss consultants are the primary reasons to visit Green Valley. They also offer Native American and Shaman healing rituals and an Alternative Healing Center.

The Hills Health & Guest Ranch
British Columbia, Canada

Come and experience Canada's first year-round spa resort, featuring luxurious chalet or lodge accommodations, extraordinary spa cuisine, dynamite fitness facilities, pampering treatments, and 20,000 acres of trails for hiking, horseback riding, and winter skiing! Clients choose from fitness, pampering, or weight-loss programs in the scenic splendor of "supernatural" British Columbia.

Lake Austin Spa Resort
Texas

You'll feel relaxed, revived, and refreshed after a week at Lake Austin, the ultimate getaway with a "summer camp" feel, located on the beautiful shores of Lake Austin on the Colorado River. And just like the good ole camp days, you'll go home with a few new friends. This dynamite fitness resort, a well-kept secret among its devoted clientele, offers outstanding speaker programs, a friendly and personal staff, great exercise facilities and outdoor sports, pampering treatments, organically grown healthy food, plenty of tranquillity, and a lot of fun!

Rancha La Puerta
Baja California, Mexico

At Rancha La Puerta, the day begins at dawn for those who want to climb the sage-scented trails of sacred Mount Kuchumaa, or welcome the sun in an open-air pavilion. Devote your days to an exciting, life-changing fitness program, selecting classes from the more than fifty offered; feast on delicious spa cuisine (an organic garden has been an integral part of the ranch since its founding fifty-four years ago); pamper yourself in the new beauty center; or discover your mind, body, and spirit in the spectacular new gym.

Safety Harbor Resort
Florida

Safety Harbor is certainly the resort that has it all: dynamic classes, soothing treatments, fabulous food, tennis courts, a golf course...you name it. Whether you're looking for the all-natural Clarins skin-care program, a personalized exercise program, sports training, or Phil Green's Tennis Academy, you're in the right hands. The facilities have been enhanced by a recent multimillion dollar renovation to the bedrooms, dining room, and spa. Their highlights include outstanding water exercise and new tranquil fitness classes.

Westglow Spa
North Carolina

This exquisitely furnished mansion in the mountains of North Carolina has the feeling of a super-romantic B&B, filled with priceless antiques, objets d'art, and surrounded by the most glorious views. Westglow is also the home of a state-of-the-art spa, with great fitness facilities and luxurious spa treatments.

Luxury

Cal-A-Vie
California

This most elegant of spa retreats in the hill country north of San Diego, Cal-A-Vie resembles a small village in Provence. Each glorious day begins with a walk through verdant hills, followed by breakfast served on beautiful linens and lovely china. Classes include aerobics, step aerobics, body contour, weight training, boxercise with a championship trainer, and water exercise. Afternoons, guests willingly surrender to a heavenly regime of treatments. Lunch and dinner offer tantalizing dishes from the chef's extraordinary repertoire, enjoyed with friendly talk among the guests. This luxurious program runs every week from Sunday to Saturday.

Golden Door
California

Created amid the undisturbed natural beauty of an oak-shaded canyon near San Diego, the Golden Door embodies the vision of its dynamic founder, Deborah Szekely. Inspired by her travels, she built a stunning replica of a Japanese honjin inn, with its centuries-old tradition of providing the most thoughtful care. No other spa has so perfectly captured the imagination of its guests and consistently surpassed their expectations. The world's finest year-round climate, one-on-one fitness training, extraordinary cuisine, attention to detail, utmost tranquillity. . . all combine for top spa value at an all-inclusive price. The Golden Door is exclusively for women, except for a few weeks that are co-ed or for men only.

The Greenhouse
Texas

Celebrating its thirtieth birthday, the Greenhouse has remained among the elite of the spa industry because of its unique philosophy and unwavering attention to detail. Twice distinguished as providing the "Best in Spa Cuisine" by readers of *Condé Nast Traveler* and

"Best Accommodations/Facilities," the Greenhouse is unsurpassed in its culinary excellence and luxurious environment. The Greenhouse is also renowned for providing the finest in state-of-the-art fitness, beauty, and massage programs—each custom-tailored to help patrons achieve their individual goals. Programs run from Sunday to Sunday, exclusively for women.

Miraval, Life in Balance
Arizona

In the high desert of southern Arizona, there's a place where you can learn to manage the pressures of daily life, a new kind of luxury spa resort called Miraval. You can enjoy a program especially created to meet your goals for stress management, relaxation, and self-discovery, while you experience all of the pleasures of incomparable service and amenities. Choose from an uncommon variety of enjoyable activities, each offering you specific ways to lead a healthier, happier life. You'll take home more than memories—you'll leave with a genuine sense of well-being and proven stress reduction techniques.

Behavior Modification and Weight Management

Green Mountain at Fox Run
Vermont

A program for women who understand that weight loss means not only changing your relationship with food, but also permanently changing your behavior. While you learn how to eat well, exercise, and manage stress, the supportive professional team helps you develop a personalized "take-home" program that will ensure long-term success. This acclaimed women's program boasts the highest long-term success rate in the nation. Of course, being in Vermont makes it even more special.

Hilton Head Health Institute
South Carolina

On a beautiful subtropical barrier sea island, with miles and miles of white sandy beach, you'll find this famous health education center, specializing in the promotion of good health, habit change, and weight control. Dr. Peter Miller, the founder and its executive director, is a clinical psychologist and the internationally acclaimed author of many best-selling books. His staff is extremely supportive and committed to the participants' success.

Structure House
North Carolina

Structure House is a great place to lose weight, develop healthy long-term habits, and enjoy rejuvenating exercise. The focus of their program is behavioral, with an emphasis on clients' relationships with food. Participants learn to identify and understand the

antecedents of eating for non-nutritional reasons and develop resources and coping strategies to make successful changes at home.

Spas on a Budget

Birdwing Spa
Minnesota

On this 300-acre estate of beautiful country, resplendent with lakes, forest, and prairie, guests are free to take it all in, or just take it easy. Fill your days with revitalizing exercise, healthful dining, and unabashed pampering, and your evenings with country serenity. The intimate atmosphere makes for a unique experience.

Fit for Life
Florida

At this fabulous spa resort on its own beautiful stretch of white sand beach, you can enjoy the purely vegetarian lifestyle, let go of stress, participate in fitness classes, and listen to valuable lectures on health by the resident medical director and natural health practitioner.

Franklin Quest Institute of Fitness
Utah

In the beautiful red rock canyon of southern Utah, this spa has become known for its incredible value and its repeated success in the fields of weight loss and physical fitness. It's the perfect place to regain your health, relax, and eliminate stress.

Hosteria Las Quintas
Morelos, Mexico

Guests can explore the Mexican countryside and history through the fabulous eco-fitness programs, or spend hours at the spa being soothed, pampered, and spoiled with a variety of expert skin and body treatments. Other amenities include: spa dining at your choice of restaurants, the glorious golf courses of Cuernevaca, a fitness gym, yoga classes, and plenty of opportunity for bargain and treasure hunting at local markets.

Ixtapan Resort and Spa
Mexico

Whether you want to relax, lose weight, or participate in sports, Ixtapan Resort and Spa provides extra value in the number of treatments and activities available. You can even brush up on your game of tennis or golf (lessons included) in this idyllic climate in the heart of the Sierra Madre Mountains in Colonial Mexico.

The Palms
California

Visit the Palms and you'll see why fitness-minded vacationers come here year-round. One price includes three spa cuisine meals a day, choice of fourteen fun-filled daily fitness classes (including stretching and water aerobics), and unlimited personal attention from a dedicated staff of experts.

Resorts with Spa Programs

Doral Golf Resort & Spa
Florida

The spa at Doral is recognized as one of the world's most luxurious, featuring relaxing European spa treatments, a versatile fitness program for all levels, gourmet spa cuisine, and all the amenities of the adjacent Doral Golf Resort. Ideal for singles and couples, the spa at Doral offers forty-eight luxurious suites, each with private balcony, Jacuzzi, and entertainment center. Programs include pampering, stress management, weight loss, and cellulite reduction. All four- and seven-night programs also include limousine transfers to and from Miami International Airport.

La Costa Resort & Spa
California

This world-class European-style spa resort has been one of the leading spas in the United States for over twenty-five years, offering a wide variety of programs and packages. Massages, facials, manicures, pedicures, aromatherapy, body wraps, and hydrotherapy baths are just some of the services provided. You'll also find lavish accommodations, championship golf courses, and exquisite dining options (including spa cuisine); La Costa is definitely not for those who want to rough it!

The Peaks
Colorado
Perched high atop the southern Colorado Rockies, this luxury spa resort is the ideal escape. Magnificent views, pure mountain air, and an astounding 42,000-square-foot spa facility (with forty-four treatment rooms!) offer anything under the sun, from state-of-the-art fitness to relaxing, soothing, purifying, and restorative treatments.

The Phoenician
Arizona
High in the beautiful Sonoran desert, you'll find the stunning and ultra-luxurious Phoenician resort, complete with a golf course, tennis courts, and The Centre for Well-Being. Inspired by the balance and serenity of the surrounding desert, the Centre offers dozens of ways to renew and invigorate your body, mind, and spirit. This spectacular facility is home to a full array of spa services, including steam, sauna, whirlpool, Swiss showers, aerobic and weight training studios, and a meditation atrium. Special programs are available for children.

Solace Spa at Banff Springs Hotel
Alberta, Canada
This spectacular hotel, designed on a truly grand scale, is located within the boundaries of the National Park. There is astonishing scenery and abundant wildlife—share the fairway with elk, deer, or foxes; catch a glimpse of eagles and bighorn sheep while you ski or hike. The Solace Spa, with its spectacular skylight, cascading waterfalls, and comfortable lounges, is not only a place to get fit, active, and expertly spoiled, but it's also a fabulous place to do absolutely nothing.

Adventure

Global Fitness Adventures
Imagine yourself enjoying daily eight- to eighteen-mile scenic wilderness hikes (geared to fit your fitness ability and pace); afternoon horseback riding; yoga, Tai Chi, meditation, and muscle toning classes; mountain biking; whitewater rafting; and three massages a week. Inspiring evening programs include motivational talks on nutrition and longevity, personal power and mind mapping, drumming and dance workshops, and Indian sweat lodges. Stay in an upscale, private estate home on a beautiful 1,500-acre horse and llama ranch where a private chef prepares delicious, healthy food.

Other scheduled trips available: Santa Barbara, California; Dominica, Caribbean; Bali; Bhutan or Nepal; and Spa-Fari in Kenya. *For corporate or custom trips for six or more people they also offer:* Santa Cruz Island, California; St. John, Caribbean; Mount Shasta, California; Careyes, Mexico; Lake Como, Italy; and Devonshire, England.

Suggested Reading

I don't just love writing books. . . I love reading them, too! The ones I've listed below are just some of the books that have inspired and educated me. But don't limit yourself to this list—head to your local bookstore and start browsing.

Ageless Body, Timeless Mind
DEEPAK CHOPRA, M.D.
(Harmony Books)
Deepak Chopra combines modern medicine with current antiaging research to reveal how the effects of aging are largely preventable. By intervening at the level where belief becomes biology, this book will show you how to achieve your unbounded potential, providing readers with the tools to create new perceptions of aging, harness the power of awareness, and experience a sense of timelessness.

All That She Can Be
DR. CAROL EAGLE AND CAROL COLMAN
(Simon & Schuster)
This books offers sound, comprehensive advice on how to avert the well-known precipitous drop in self-esteem that American girls typically experience as they become teenagers.

All Things are Possible—Pass the Word
BARBARA MILO OHRBACH
(Clarkson Potter)
A small gift book filled with positive, lively quotations that emphasize a can-do approach to life and all of its wonderful possibilities. Encouraging and empowering, inspiring and comforting, it's the ideal gift for someone you care about.

The Can-Do Eating Plan for Overweight Kids and Teens
MICHELLE DAUM
(Avon Books)
This terrific book is designed to help kids control their weight, look better, and feel great. Michelle Daum's revolutionary program is easy to follow and really works.

Dr. Nancy Snyderman's Guide to Good Health
NANCY L. SNYDERMAN, M.D.
(William Morrow & Co.)
This terrific book provides facts that every woman over forty should know about her changing body and changing health, from *GMA* medical correspondent Dr. Nancy Snyderman.

Find a Quiet Corner
NANCY O'HARA
(Warner Books)
This book will help keep you from rushing through your day, draining yourself of energy and increasing your level of stress. Going beyond simple daily meditations, *Find a Quiet Corner* teaches you how to unwind, experience a new infusion of energy, and get in touch with your own reservoir of strength and calmness. You'll discover how to tap into these resources and enter your own private sanctum at any time.

Fit Over Forty
JAMES M. RIPPE, M.D.
(William Morrow & Co.)
This is a book that offers hope and a new vision of health and fitness, as well as a revolutionary approach to achieving total well-being and personal peace, for people in their forties. The author is one of America's leading cardiologists, an authority on health and fitness, and a regular guest on GMA. This

book is based on a yearlong scientific study that established the first-ever comprehensive fitness standards by age and sex for people over forty. It provides specific information and a concrete fitness program for anyone at this stage in his or her life.

Fodor's Healthy Escapes
BERNARD BURT
(Fodor's Travel Publications, Inc.)
A complete guide to 243 resorts and retreats where you can get fit, feel good, find yourself, and get away from it all.

Full Catastrophe Living
JON KABAT-ZINN, PH.D.
(Delta Books)
This book teaches you how to use the wisdom of your body and mind to counteract stress, pain, and illness.

Healing Mind, Healthy Woman
ALICE D. DOMAR, PH.D., AND HENRY DREHER
(Henry Holt & Co.)
This book teaches you how to use the mind-body connection to manage stress and take control of your life. It offers a new repertoire of therapeutic methods to two broad groups of women—those who wish to maintain their good health and those who are suffering from specific health problems. Dr. Domar describes a spectrum of techniques for stress management and wellness for all women. Each chapter contains stories of women who have

achieved remarkable success in Dr. Domar's programs, proving that you can use the mind-body connection to seize control of your health and well-being.

Joan Lunden's Healthy Cooking
JOAN LUNDEN AND LAURA MORTON
(Little, Brown and Company)
This book is part cookbook, part inspirational story on how I've lost and kept off more than fifty pounds, with over one hundred recipes that are easy to prepare, delicious, healthy, and nutritious.

Journey Into Healing
DEEPAK CHOPRA, M.D.
(Harmony Books)
A selection of essential thoughts from Deepak Chopra's other books, taking readers through the experience of a journey into healing. The passages are meant to influence your perceptions and mobilize your body's natural tendency toward perfect health. The book's purpose is to awaken the wisdom that already exists within you.

Make the Connection
BOB GREENE AND OPRAH WINFREY
(Hyperion)
Oprah Winfrey and her personal trainer, Bob Greene, show you exactly what to do every day, physically and mentally, to begin looking and feeling great. They provide a fitness program that's easy to follow, along with inspiring personal stories.

The Menopause Book
SHELDON H. CHERRY, M.D. AND
CAROLYN D. RUNOWICZ, M.D.
(Macmillan Publishing)
A guide to health and well being for women over forty, *The Menopause Book* skillfully blends science and personal experience to define and describe menopause and discuss related issues. Women who are about to enter menopause will learn how to recognize the signs of its onset, to determine which symptoms are normal, and to relieve any discomfort they may esperience.

Meditations
EKNATH EASWARAN
(Nilgiri Press)
A simple eight-step program for incorporating spiritual ideals into daily life.

Meditations for Women Who Do Too Much
ANNE WILSON SCHAEF
(HarperCollins)
This book gathers quotes from women all over the world and combines them with wise daily meditations for any woman who wants to slow down for a minute and make time for herself—to laugh a little, share a moment of inspiration, and remind herself that she's worth taking care of.

The Meditative Mind
DANIEL GOLEMAN
(Tarcher/Putnam)
This book is an excellent source for readers who wonder about the different varieties of meditation and the meditative experience. Written with depth, authority, and understanding, it's a great avenue for spiritual seekers to explore and understand the supermarket of spiritual practices now available.

Minding Your Body
JOSEPH S. RECHTSCHAFFEN, M.D. AND ROBERT CAROLA
(HarperCollins)
With an emphasis on the power your mind can have over your body, this book offers practical advice and useful information on subjects such as stress, exercise, vitamins, and positive thinking.

The Modern Woman's Guide to Life
ELIZABETH CHAPMAN, MARGARET KASSNER, AND KAREN KRIBERNEY
(Harper & Row)
If you really want help solving some of life's more day-to-day problems, this book has the answers. It covers everything from cars to careers and clothing to carpentry, and is a must-have handbook for every modern woman.

Power Foods
LIZ APPLEGATE, PH.D.
High-performance nutrition for high-performance people is the premise of this book, which teaches you how to fuel your body for success. It's filled with hundreds of ideas on how to punch up your performance at the gym and on the job, and helpful tips on how to incorporate healthy eating into any lifestyle.

Practical Intuition
LAURA DAY
(Villard Books)
This book will teach you to harness the power of your instinct and make it work for you. Laura Day's techniques can be used to unlock the remarkable powers of your mind and help you make decisions about every facet of your life.

Quantum Leap Thinking
JAMES J. MAPES
(Dove)
Consider this book an owner's manual for your mind. It's an extraordinary guide to thinking your way to the next level in your life, within your career, your relationships, or your self. You'll learn how to implement positive change and make quantum leaps in your personal growth, by defining your vision and developing a road map to get you there. The book also offers strategies, insights, practical exercises, and advice to help you build a personal support system around you.

Reviving Ophelia: Saving the Selves of Adolescent Girls
MARY PIPHER, PH.D.
(G.P. Putnam's Sons)
This book takes an eye-opening look at the dangers of everyday life for adolescent girls. Based on actual cases she has treated, Dr. Pipher offers much-needed advice to parents of teenage girls on how to help their daughters grow into healthy adults with strength, self esteem, and positive self images. Told through the voices of the girls themselves, their stories are powerful, personal, and painfully honest. The girls reveal how they've fallen prey to depression, eating disorders, addictions, and suicidal urges, all at a much higher rate than twenty years ago. This book is a must-read for parents with daughters.

Rituals for the Bath
KATHY COREY AND LYNNE BLACKMAN
(Warner Treasures)
This book will inspire you to reconnect with the glories of bathing, and to create natural bath products that are as simple to make as they are indulgent. Easy, inexpensive recipes and basic instructions will help you make other unusual gift items.

Secrets of Inner Peace
J. DONALD WALTERS
(Crystal Clarity)
With a seed of thought for every day of the month, this little handbook is filled with inspirational ideas that, if practiced regularly, can become an integral part of your normal consciousness.

Seven Keys to Vibrant Health
TERRY LEMEROND
(Impakt Communication)
This book provides a simple method to living a healthier, happier, longer, more painless life. Each chapter offers new ways to obtain optimum health and follows a detailed blueprint to achieving lasting health in all realms, from financial to spiritual.

Sleep Thieves
STANLEY COREN
(Free Press/Simon & Schuster)
An eye-opening exploration into the science and mysteries of the A to ZZZ's of sleep. Author Stanley Coren provides astounding new evidence that we are becoming an increasingly sleep-deprived society and reveals the potential dangers of this condition

Surfing the Himalayas
FREDERICK LENZ
(St. Martin's Press)
One of the only fictional books on my list, this book tells the story of a young snowboarder who travels through the Himalayas in search of the ultimate high, only to surf into an experience more transcendent than he ever imagined. The young snowboarder meets a Buddhist monk who teaches him that by freeing his mind and challenging his soul, he can master any mountain.

Timeless Healing

HERBERT BENSON, M.D., with MARG STARK

(Scribner)

Dr. Benson illustrates his theory on the power and biology of belief. He explores the intersection between objective science and the mystifying power of the human spirit to reveal how affirming beliefs—particularly belief in a higher power—make a critical contribution to our physical health.

When Feeling Bad Is Good

ELLEN MCGRATH, PH.D.

(Henry Holt)

Written by *GMA* correspondent Ellen McGrath, this is a practical, user-friendly book that shows women how to achieve greater independence, health, and well-being, and a guide to converting "healthy" depression into new sources of growth and power.

Wherever You Go, There You Are

JON KABAT-ZINN, PH.D.

(Hyperion)

This book is a remarkably clear and practical guide to meditation and wakefulness. Jon Kabat-Zinn maps out a simple path for cultivating mindfulness and reclaiming the richness of life's moments, for people just coming into meditation, as well as longtime practitioners.

A Woman's Guide to a Simpler Life

ANDREA VAN STEENHOUSE, PH.D.

(Harmony Books)

A thoughtful primer on clearing your head as well as your closets, this book reveals the three main obstacles to simplifying your life. You'll learn how to make space for what is truly of value in your life—family, work, home, and friendships—through useful advice and anecdotes.

Women's Bodies, Women's Wisdom

CHRISTIANE NORTHRUP, M.D.

(Bantam Books)

In this book on maintaining good physical and emotional health through holistic medicine, Christiane Northrup combines curing with caring and knowledge with intuition to demonstrate how physical healing and spiritual healing are inseparable.

Internet Options

One of the best resource bookstores in the country for health and self-help books is the Bodhi Tree in Los Angeles. They offer a newsletter and a very complete catologue of titles. The store is also affiliated with a new Internet website named Health World Online—A Comprehensive Alternative Healthcare Center. The Health World Online address is: **http://www.healthy.net**. Bodhi Tree is the official bookstore for the website, offering a complete selection of materials. The direct Internet address for the Bodhi Tree is: **http://www.healthy.net/market/book**. They are also at e-mail address: **bodhitree@bodhitree.com** for all non-Health World Online orders and requests.

Index

Index

Negative thinking; Power thinking; Stress; *specific emotions*
Endurance training, 32, 227–31
Energy foods, 211–15
Estrogen replacement, 234
Evans, Scot, 36, 82–83, 99, 149
Exercise, 55, 88, 109, 216–31
  benefits of, 216–17
  for better bones, 231–34
  drinking water and, 207–8
  eating before, 215
  finding time for, 219–20
  maximizing efficiency of, 222–23
  mental attitude and, 218–19
  metabolic benefits of, 225–26
  newlyweds and, 181
  older population and, 54–55, 198, 200–201
  personal goals for, 221–22
  for strength and endurance, 227–31
  for teenagers, 171
  See also Weight training
Expectations, 86

Family of choice, 195–96
Fat, dietary, 166, 208–9
Fear, 87
Fiber, 209, 233
Fifties (age), 84, 193–94
Fit for Life, Florida, 244
Fit Over Forty (Rippe), 187, 194, 249
Food. *See* Dieting; Eating disorders; Nutrition
Food addiction, 178
Forties (age), 83–84, 188–93, 216
Franklin Quest Institute of Fitness (Florida), 244
Free Willy 2 (film), 60
Friends, 119, 201
Fruits, 209
Fruit Smoothie, 213
Frustration, 85
Fun, importance of, 72

Getting Your Kids to Say "No" in the Nineties (Strasburger), 175, 249
Gibson, Charlie, 13, 93
Global Fitness Adventures, 246
Goals, setting, 63, 65–66, 88, 113–14

Golden Door Spa (California), 24–30, 99, 243
Good Morning America (TV program), 13, 91–93, 96–97, 136
  and Disney/ABC News, 154–55, 157–58
  health series, 19–21
  spoofs of, 92
Gottman, John, 181
Grand Teton Chicken Noodle Soup, 44
Grand Tetons (Wyoming), 37–51
Great American Back Rub Stores, 145
Greene, Bob, 54, 250
The Greenhouse (Texas), 243
Green Mountain at Fox Run (Vermont), 243–44
Green Valley Spa (Utah), 241
Grudges, 85–86
Guilt, 109–10
Gynecologists, 169, 171

Happiness, 75–77, 108–9
Hartman, David, 92
Hawn, Goldie, 84, 136, 193–94
Headaches, 211
Healing Mind, Healthy Woman (Domar and Dreher), 116, 249–50
Health and healing
  balance in life affecting, 54–57
  exercise and, 216–31
  life cycles and, 165–201
  optimism affecting, 105–6
Health resorts, 241–46
Heart disease, 54, 187, 200, 216
Heart rate, 223–25
  cardiovascular capacity, 32
Higher road, 82–83, 103, 127
The Hills Health & Guest Ranch (British Columbia), 241
Hilton Head Health Institute (South Carolina), 244
Hormone (estrogen) replacement, 234
Hosteria Las Quintas (Mexico)245

Ibuprophen, 173
Imposter phenomenon, 175
Inactivity, 54
Inspirational books and messages, 113

Internet options, 255
Ixapan Resort and Spa (Mexico), 245

Jackson Hole (Wyoming), 37
Jamie (author's daughter), 68, 71, 72, 74, 75, 141
  health issues and, 166–68, 171
  pink hair and, 125–26
  writing and, 99, 167–68
Jamison, Robert, 144
Jet lag, 237
Joan Lunden's Healthy Cooking (Lunden and Morton), 250
Job market, 178–79
Johnson, Barbara, 199
Johnson, Jay, 12–13
Johnson, Jed, 12–14, 15
Johnson, Tim, 204, 233
Journey Into Healing (Lunden and Morton), 250
Judgmental behavior, 87

Kabat-Zinn, Jon, 85, 87, 123–24, 147, 154, 249, 254
Kaehler, Kathy, 151
Kalish, Susan, 207
Knutson, Steve, 48
Kranin, Ralph, 130–31
Krieger, Ellie, 207, 213, 215
Kutner, Lawrence, 184

La Costa Resort & Spa (California), 245
Lake, Ricki, 51–53
Lake Austin Spa Resort (Texas), 242
Lake Placid Horse Show, 72
La Palestra (New York City), 30–36, 37
Laxatives, 233
Learned Optimism (Seligman), 109
Letting go, 85–87, 101, 103
Life cycles, 165–201
  age fifty, 193–94
  age forty, 188–93
  golden years, 196–201
  love/marriage and, 179–81
  menstrual cycle and, 171–73
  pregnancy/motherhood and, 182–88
  teenage years, 166–78
  See also Aging

Index